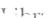

Get Through
MRCPsych Parts 1 and 2: 1001 EMIQs

Editor

Albert Michael MBBS MD DPM MRCPsych

Consultant in Adult Psychiatry
West Suffolk Hospital, UK

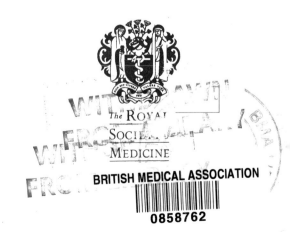

© 2004 Royal Society of Medicine Ltd

Reprinted 2006

Published by the Royal Society of Medicine Press Ltd
1 Wimpole Street, London W1G 0AE, UK
Tel: +44 (0)20 7290 2921
Fax: +44 (0)20 7290 2929
E-mail: publishing@rsm.ac.uk
Website: www.rsmpress.co.uk

British Library Cataloguing in Publication Data
A catalogue record for this book is available from the British Library

ISBN: 1-85315-599-3

Distribution in Europe and Rest of the World:

Marston Book Services Ltd
PO Box 269
Abingdon
Oxon OX14 4YN, UK
Tel: +44 (0)1235 465500
Fax: +44 (0)1235 465666

Distribution in USA and Canada:

Royal Society of Medicine Press Ltd
c/o JAMCO Distribution Inc
1401 Lakeway Drive
Lewisville, TX 75057, USA
Tel: +1 800 538 1287
Fax: +1 972 353 1303
E-mail: jamco@majors.com

Distribution in Australia and New Zealand:

Elsevier Australia
30–52 Smidmore Street
Marrikville NSW 2204, Australia
Tel: +61 2 9517 8999
Fax: +61 2 9517 2249
E-mail: service@elsevier.com.au

Phototypeset by Phoenix Photosetting, Chatham, Kent
Printed in the UK by Bell & Bain Ltd, Glasgow

Contents

Foreword

I am a firm believer in the idea that a good examination teaches more than it tests, so long as the candidate is thoroughly prepared; the teaching, learning, revision and examination together form an educational package. This excellent book will do as it says it will. It will help people prepare for the Membership Examination of the Royal College of Psychiatrists, that considerable hurdle before candidates can undertake higher training in clinical psychiatry and continue their professional life.

Dr Michael has drawn on his considerable experience in organising the highly successful Cambridge Course for the MRCPsych that has had above average pass rates under the previous and new syllabuses; teaching for the objective structured clinical examination (OSCE) and the extended matching item questions (EMIQs) is now well established. Many experts, ex-students and colleagues who contribute to that course have devised an extensive set of EMIQs that cover the entire range of subjects and concepts that are required by the examination and that underpin our discipline; two hundred bases are covered. For those of us who won't get everything correct at the first attempt, working through the questions, perhaps having first tried them under exam conditions, will lead us to textbooks, lecture notes and other sources that will emphasise common principles as well as leading us towards novel and rarely explored facts. Students and their teachers, as well as anyone interested in or practising psychiatry will enjoy the results of this effort.

In their review of the new examination and the reasons for change, Tyrer and Oyebode comment that the MRCPsych is, "in educational parlance, a high-stakes examination". Most candidates will not have needed to consult a learned journal to come to that view, though I recommend that they read the article so as to understand more about why the examination has developed into its present form. Most candidates will, however, be helped by working through the 1001 questions in this book. Many will have much to thank Dr Michael for when that fateful envelope falls onto the doormat bearing their results and, thereafter, as their studies continue during their professional lives. Good luck!

Peter B. Jones
Professor of Psychiatry
University of Cambridge

REFERENCE

1. Tyrer S, Oyebode F. Why does the MRCPsych examination need to change? Br J Psychiatry 2004; 184: 197–99.

Preface

The EMIQs were introduced into the MRCPsych exams in 2003. EMIQs form one-third of the theory exam in the Part I and a lesser proportion in the Part II theory exams.

Why EMIQs? The Individual Statement Questions have only two possible answers, i.e. 'True' or 'False', hence they test only rote memory and not reasoning. The EMIQs, on the other hand, by providing a greater range of options, test in-depth knowledge, logical thinking, reasoning and judgement. The EMIQ situation is more akin to how clinicians think in their clinical practise.

EMIQs are here to stay.

SOURCES OF FURTHER INFORMATION

Tyrer S, Oyebode F. Why does the MRCPsych examination need to change? Br J Psychiatr 2004; 184: 197–99.
http://www.cambridgecourse.com
http://www.prepdublin.com
http://www.rcpsych.ac.uk
http://www.superego-café.com
http://www.trickcyclists.co.uk

Contributors

Regi T Alexander MRCPsych
Consultant Psychiatrist
St John's House Hospital
Diss
Norfolk, UK

Jennifer Anderson BSc (Hons), MBBS, MRCPsych
Specialist Registrar in Psychiatry
Cambridge, UK

Chittaranjan Andrade MD
Additional Professor
Department of Psychopharmacology
National Institute of Mental Health and Neurosciences
Bangalore, India

Claire Dibben MRCPsych
Specialist Registrar in Psychiatry
Cambridge, UK

Vinu George MD
Department of Psychiatry
Albert Einstein Medical Center
Philadelphia, PA
USA

Maju Mathews MD, MRCPsych, DPM
Department of Psychiatry
Drexel University College of Medicine
Philadelphia, PA
USA

Manu Mathews MD
Department of Psychiatry
Cleveland Clinic Foundation
Cleveland, OH
USA

Albert Michael MBBS, MD, DPM, MRCPsych
Consultant in Adult Psychiatry
West Suffolk Hospital
Bury St Edmunds
Suffolk, UK

Graham Murray MRCPsych
Clinical Lecturer
Department of Psychiatry
University of Cambridge
Cambridge, UK

Chris O'Loughlin MRCP, MRCPsych
Specialist Registrar in Psychiatry
Assistant Organiser, Cambridge MRCPsych Course
Cambridge, UK

Brian Parsons MICGP MRCPsych
Senior Registrar in Psychiatry
National Hire Training
Scheme in Psychiatry
Ireland

Radhika Ramkumar MBBS, MRCPsych
Specialist Registrar in Psychiatry of Learning Disabilities
North West London
London, UK

Michael Robertson MB BS, FRANZCP
Director
Mayo-Wesley Centre for Mental Health
Taree, Australia

Michael D Spencer MA MB MRCPsych
Clinical Lecturer
Department of Psychiatry
University of Edinburgh
Edinburgh, UK

Nishrin B Spencer MA MB MRCP
Specialist Registrar in Renal Medicine
Edinburgh Royal Infirmary
Edinburgh, UK

Paul Wilkinson MA MB BChir DCH MRCPsych
Specialist Registrar in Child and Adolescent Psychiatry
Cambridge, UK

List of EMIQs

1. History
1.1 Abuse of psychiatry: Michael Robertson
1.2 Concepts: Michael Robertson
1.3 Contemporary researchers: Chittaranjan Andrade
1.4 History of psychiatry: Chittaranjan Andrade
1.5 History of schizophrenia Chittaranjan Andrade

2. Psychology
2.1 Concepts in learning theory: Vinu George
2.2 Defence mechanisms: Chittaranjan Andrade
2.3 Developmental stages: Albert Michael
2.4 Ego defence mechanisms: Albert Michael
2.5 Emotions: Albert Michael
2.6 Human development: Albert Michael
2.7 Illness: Albert Michael
2.8 Learning: Albert Michael
2.9 Learning theory: Maju Mathews
2.10 Memory: Albert Michael
2.11 Psychological trauma: Michael Robertson

3. Psychopathology
3.1 Affective states: Claire Dibben
3.2 Catatonic symptoms: Albert Michael
3.3 Defence mechanism and disorders: Albert Michael
3.4 Delusions: Albert Michael
3.5 Disorders of perception: Albert Michael
3.6 First-rank symptoms: Albert Michael
3.7 Formal thought disorder: Albert Michael
3.8 Obsessions: Albert Michael
3.9 Psychopathology: Michael Robertson
3.10 Symptoms: Albert Michael
3.11 Thought disorder: Albert Michael

4. Neurosciences
4.1 Agnosias and apraxias: Chris O'Loughlin
4.2 Eye signs: Radhika Ramkumar
4.3 Functional neuroanatomy: Graham Murray
4.4 Glial cells: Albert Michael
4.5 Neuroanatomical localisation: Graham Murray
4.6 Neuroanatomical regions: Graham Murray
4.7 Neuropathology of dementias: Brian Parsons
4.8 Pathophysiology: Michael Robertson
4.9 Pathophysiology of schizophrenia: Graham Murray

5. Assessment and classification
5.1 Aetiological factors: Maju Mathews
5.2 Aetiology: Graham Murray
5.3 Aetiology of dementias: Brian Parsons

I. History

1.1   Abuse of psychiatry

Options

a. Ankangs
b. Deep sleep therapy
c. Execution of mentally retarded
d. Hiroshima
e. Homosexuality
f. Operation T4
g. The Serbsky Institute
h. Tuskegee Study
i. Unit 371
j. Hendrik Verwoerd

Lead in

Match the historical abuse of psychiatry with its common reference term:

Historical abuses

1. Nazi-era psychiatry
2. Soviet-era psychiatry
3. Apartheid-era psychiatry
4. Deliberate denial of treatment for African Americans with syphilis
5. Repression of Falun Gong

1.2   Concepts

Options

a. Being and Time
b. Beyond the Pleasure Principle
c. Le Suicide
d. Loss
e. Madness and Civilization
f. Persuasion and Healing
g. Talking to Prozac
h. The Ailment
i. The Asylum
j. The Divided Self

Lead in

Match the following concepts with the works above:

Concepts

1. Negative countertransference
2. Thanatos
3. Ontology
4. Anomia
5. Healing agent

1.3 Contemporary researchers

Options

a. Community psychiatry
b. Drug trials
c. Eating disorder
d. Electroconvulsive therapy
e. Mood disorders
f. Neuroimaging in schizophrenia
g. Neuropsychiatry
h. Personality disorders
i. Psychopharmacology
j. Transcultural psychiatry

Lead in

Match one area each with the following researchers:

Researchers

1. Stephen Stahl
2. Hagop Akiskal
3. Harold Sackeim
4. John Kane
5. Michael Trimble

1.4 History of psychiatry

Options

a. Introduction of lithium
b. Introduction of chlorpromazine
c. Introduction of imipramine
d. Introduction of electroconvulsive therapy (ECT)
e. Genetics of schizophrenia
f. Family studies on schizophrenia
g. Nosology of schizophrenia
h. Nosology of bipolar disorder
i. Cognitive behaviour therapy (CBT)
j. Group psychotherapy

Lead in

Match one option each with the following pairs of researchers:

Researchers

1. Vaughn and Leff
2. Krauthammer and Klerman
3. Delay and Deniker
4. Cerletti and Bini
5. Gottesman and Shields

1.5   History of schizophrenia

Options

a. Andreasen
b. Bleuler
c. Cade
d. Freud
e. Goodwin
f. Hoch and Polatin
g. Kasanin
h. Langfeldt
i. Mayer-Gross
j. Morel

Lead in

Match one option each with the following terms/concepts in relation to schizophrenia:

Terms/Concepts

1. Schizoaffective psychosis
2. Oneirophrenia
3. Pseudoneurotic schizophrenia
4. Process schizophrenia
5. Splitting

Answers

1.1 Abuse of psychiatry

1-f. Operation T4, after the HQ of the program Tiergartenstrasse 4.
2-g. The Serbsky Institute in Moscow was the focus of Soviet era psychiatry.
3-j. Hendrik Verwoerd, a psychologist was one-time leader of South Africa and used psychiatric grounds to help craft Apartheid.
4-h. The Tuskegee study attempted a naturalistic follow up of syphilis in Black Americans through denial of treatment. President Clinton eventually apologized on behalf of the US Government.
5-a. Ankangs are secure psychiatric hospitals in China where Falun Gong 'dissidents' are 'treated' for the mysterious 'quijong related mental disorder'.

1.2 Concepts

1-h. The Ailment.
2-b. Beyond the Pleasure Principle.
3-j. The Divided Self.
4-c. Le Suicide.
5-f. Persuasion and Healing.

1.3 Contemporary researchers

1-i. Psychopharmacology.
2-e. Mood disorders.
3-d. ECT, especially stimulus dosing and electrode placement.
4-b. Drug trials, especially, the 1988 study which led to the reintroduction of clozapine.
5-g. Neuropsychiatry.

1.4 History of psychiatry

1-f. Family studies on schizophrenia, especially expressed emotions and their influence on the risk of relapse in patients with schizophrenia.
2-h. Nosology of bipolar disorder, especially the concept of secondary mania.
3-b. Introduction of chlorpromazine, in 1952.
4-d. Introduction of ECT, in 1938.
5-e. Genetics of schizophrenia, especially twin studies.

1.5 History of schizophrenia

1-g. Kasanin (1933) introduced the concept of schizoaffective illness.

2-i. Mayer-Gross (1924) described oneirophrenia as an acute form of illness, characterised by a dream-like state.

3-f. Hoch and Polatin (1949) described pseudoneurotic schizophrenia as a state of pan-anxiety, pan-neurosis, and pan-sexuality; the syndrome has presently been subsumed under the rubric of borderline personality disorder.

4-h. Langfeldt (1960) distinguished between reactive and process schizophrenia (CPS7-391).

5-b. Bleuler (1912) described schizophrenia as a condition characterised by splitting or schisms between thought, emotions and behaviour.

2. Psychology

2.1   Concepts in learning theory

Options

a. Classical conditioning
b. Extinction
c. Higher order conditioning
d. Operant conditioning
e. Positive reinforcement
f. Punishment
g. Reciprocal inhibition
h. Shaping
i. Stimulus discrimination
j. Stimulus generalisation

Lead in

Match one concept with each of the following situations:

Situations

1. A woman is involved in a car accident on the motorway. Although she did not get injured seriously, the accident terrified her. Now she avoids the motorway, because driving on it makes her too tense and nervous.
2. An instructor in a weight-management class awards participants points for every healthy meal they eat and every exercise session they complete. These points later result in part refunds of their class fees.
3. A puppy initially responds to lots of different people, but over time it learns to respond to only one or a few people's commands.
4. A child talks about many topics in the presence of his parents. The parents reinforce the child's talking by being attentive and responding. The child is then very keen to talk to the guests.
5. A child is learning to write. He is praised for holding the pencil correctly and then for scribbling something and later for writing something that vaguely resembles a letter.

2.2 Defence mechanisms

Options

a. Acting out
b. Denial
c. Dissociation
d. Intellectualisation
e. Isolation
f. Passive aggression
g. Projection
h. Repression
i. Sublimation
j. Suppression

Lead in

Select one ego defence mechanism each for the following descriptions:

Descriptions

1. Failure to recognise or accept conflict
2. Pushing a conflict from the conscious mind into the unconscious mind such that the conflict cannot be recalled by an act of will
3. Pushing a conflict from the conscious mind into the preconscious mind such that the conflict can be recalled by an act of will
4. Ascribing to others the unacceptable motives that lie within oneself
5. Expressing resentment by non-cooperation, forgetting, and other such means

2.3   Developmental stages

Options

a. Phallic
b. Preconventional morality
c. Preoperational
d. Puberty
e. Reward orientation
f. Sensorimotor
g. Social contract–legalistic orientation
h. The phase of symbiosis
i. Trust versus mistrust
j. Universal ethical principles orientation

Lead in

Find the stages/levels or phases of development described by the following theorists:

Theorists

1. Erikson (1)
2. Freud (1)
3. Kohlberg (3)
4. Mahler (1)
5. Piaget (2)

2.4 Ego defence mechanisms

Options

a. Acting out
b. Altruism
c. Anticipation
d. Blocking
e. Controlling
f. Denial
g. Displacement
h. Externalisation
i. Hypochondriasis
j. Inhibition

Lead in

Classify the defence mechanisms into the following groups:

Groups

1. Narcissistic (1)
2. Immature (3)
3. Neurotic (4)
4. Mature (2)

2.5 Emotions

Options

a. Cannon and Bard
b. Darwin
c. Ekman
d. Fish
e. James and Lange
f. Papez
g. Pavlov
h. Schachter–Singer cognitive labelling theory
i. Seligman
j. Skinner

Lead in

Match one term each with the following descriptions:

Descriptions

1. The perception of the emotion-arousing stimulus causes bodily changes, interpretation of which is the emotion. 'I failed, I am crying, so I must be sad'.
2. Physiological arousal (factor 1) is necessary for the experience of emotion, but the nature of arousal is immaterial – what is important is how the arousal is interpreted, i.e. the cognitive appraisal of arousal (factor 2).
3. There are six basic or primary emotions. They are universal, i.e. they are expressed facially in the same way, and are recognised as such by members of a diversity of cultures, hence they are innate.
4. The subjective emotion is quite independent of physiological changes. The thalamus processes the emotion-producing stimulus and sends the information to the cortex, where the emotion is consciously experienced, and to the hypothalamus, which sets in motion the autonomic physiological changes.
5. 'The Expression of Emotions in Man and Animals' states that particular emotional responses, e.g. facial expressions, tend to accompany the same emotional states in humans of all races and cultures, even those who are born blind.

2.6   Human development

Options

a. Anal
b. Authority orientation
c. Autistic phase
d. Autonomy versus shame and doubt
e. Concrete operations
f. Conventional morality
g. Generativity versus stagnation
h. Genital
i. Good boy–nice girl orientation
j. Identity versus role confusion

Lead in

Find the stages/levels or phases of development described by the following theorists:

Theorists

1. Erikson (3)
2. Freud (2)
3. Kohlberg (3)
4. Mahler (1)
5. Piaget (1)

2.7   Illness

Options

a. Abnormal illness behaviour
b. Adjustment disorder
c. Depression
d. Hypochondriasis
e. Illness
f. Illness behaviour
g. Sick role
h. Somatisation disorder
i. Type A behaviour
j. Type B behaviour

Lead in

Find one term each that describes the following behaviours:

Behaviours

1. Mr X, a middle-aged civil servant developed chest pains and dizziness. He felt tired and unwell.
2. He went to his doctor, had an electrocardiogram (ECG) and some blood tests. As advised by his doctor, he started a low-fat diet and doing moderate exercises.
3. His employers transferred some of his responsibilities to one of his colleagues and offered him a one-week sick leave. They were pleased to hear that he is compliant with his treatment and that he is keen to get better and to return to work as soon as possible.
4. Some of his colleagues felt that his heart problems are quite expected, considering his high ambition, driven behaviour and his tendency to be abrupt.
5. Over the next few weeks, he started feeling depressed and anxious.

2.8   Learning

Options

a. Avoidance learning
b. Classical conditioning
c. Continuous reinforcement
d. Discrimination learning
e. Experimental neurosis
f. Extinction
g. Operant conditioning
h. Reciprocal inhibition
i. Shaping
j. Stimulus generalisation

Lead in

Match one term each with the following situations:

Situations

1. A young girl used to spend a lot of time in the kitchen trying to help her mother with cooking. One day she burnt her fingers while trying to take something off the cooker. Thereafter she has been scared of going near the cooker.

2. A toddler was very scared of the new family dog. He was able to be in the same room with the dog only when he sat on his mother's lap licking his favourite ice cream.

3. Rat 'A' was moved to a cage with a lever. When the rat by chance pressed the lever, a food pellet was delivered. Food pellets were delivered every third time the rat pressed the lever. Then the rat started pressing the lever frequently.

4. Rat 'B' was moved to another cage with a number of levers. While exploring the cage, the rat accidentally pressed the different levers one after another. Food pellets were delivered only when the rat pressed one particular lever. Then the rat started pressing only the lever that delivered food.

5. Rat 'C' was moved to a new cage. When the rat walked around in certain parts of the cage but not others, it received electric shocks. Soon the rat started moving around only in the areas that were shock free.

2.9 Learning theory

Options

a. Classical conditioning
b. Discriminative learning
c. Extinction
d. Modelling
e. Operant conditioning
f. Partial reinforcement
g. Reciprocal inhibition
h. Shaping
i. Stimulus generalisation
j. Variable interval reinforcement

Lead in

Match one concept each with the following situations:

Situations

1. A rat is presented with a lever. When he accidentally presses it, food is delivered to a location below the lever. After this, the rat presses the lever further, receiving further food rewards.
2. This is the learning principle used in gambling with slot machines.
3. A child with mutism is undergoing therapy. He talks only in the presence of the therapist but not others.
4. A 12-year-old boy watches his father smoke a cigarette. He then keeps a pencil in his mouth and pretends to light it up.
5. A man with arachnophobia is told to sit in a chair and relax while listening to music and visualising pleasant and relaxing images. He is then shown a picture of a spider.

2.10 Memory

Options

a. Confabulation
b. Déjà vu
c. Jamais vu
d. Recognition
e. Recollection
f. Registration
g. Retrieval
h. Retrospective falsification
i. Semantic memory
j. Telegraphic memory

Lead in

Find one term each for the following phenomena:

Phenomena

1. The storage of information in pure form without specification of time or place.
2. The feeling of familiarity that accompanies the return of stored material to consciousness.
3. The feeling of familiarity that normally occurs with previously experienced events, occurs when the event is experienced for the first time.
4. The reintegration of a complete event from a variety of different components.
5. Modification of memories in terms of one's general attitudes.

2.11 Psychological trauma

Options

a. Primitive idealisation
b. Shattered assumptions
c. Repetition-compulsion
d. Psychological misery
e. Trauma membrane
f. Disordered self
g. Basic fault
h. Situationally accessible memory
i. Dissolution hypothesis
j. Triune brain

Lead in

Match one formulation of psychological trauma each with the following theorists:

Theorists

1. Hughlings Jackson
2. Janoff–Bullman
3. Brewin
4. Pierre Janet
5. Lindy

Answers

2.1 Concepts in learning theory

1-a. Classical conditioning (CPS7-107).
2-d. Operant conditioning. The behaviours being conditioned here are healthy eating and regular exercise. The reinforcement is the refund of the fees.
3-i. Stimulus discrimination.
4-j. Stimulus generalisation.
5-h. Shaping.

2.2. Defence mechanisms

1-b. Denial.
2-h. Repression.
3-j. Suppression.
4-g. Projection.
5-f. Passive aggression.

2.3 Developmental stages

1-i. Trust versus mistrust.
2-a. Phallic.
3-b,e,j. Preconventional morality, reward orientation, universal ethical principles orientation.
4-h. The phase of symbiosis.
5-c,f. Preoperational, sensorimotor.

2.4 Ego defence mechanisms

1-f. Denial. Also distortion; projection (CTP7-584; CPS7-314).
2-a,d,i. Acting out; blocking; hypochondriasis. Also introjection; passive-aggressive behaviour; regression; schizoid fantasy; somatisation.
3-e,g,h,j. Controlling; displacement; externalisation; inhibition. Also intellectualisation; rationalisation; dissociation; reaction formation; repression; sexualisation.
4-b,c. Altruism; anticipation. Also asceticism; humour; sublimation; suppression.

2.5 Emotions

1-e. James–Lange theory (Hilgard-396; Gross-135; CTP7-440).
2-h. Schachter–Singer cognitive labelling theory.
3-c. Ekman.
4-a. Cannon–Bard theory.
5-b. Darwin.

2.6 Human development

1-d,g,j. Erikson: Autonomy versus shame and doubt; Generativity versus stagnation, Identity versus role confusion (CTP7-610).
2-a,h. Freud: Anal, Genital (CTP7-610, 593).
3-b,f,i. Kohlberg: Authority orientation, Conventional morality, Good boy–nice girl orientation (Hilgard-86; Gross-512; CTP7-407).
4-c. Mahler: Autistic phase (CTP7-610, 593).
5-e. Piaget: Concrete operations (Gross-507; CTP7-577; NOTP-334; Hilgard-457).

2.7 Illness

1-e. Illness (OTP4-203).
2-f. Illness behaviour.
3-g. Sick role.
4-i. Type A behaviour.
5-b. Adjustment disorder.

2.8. Learning

1-b. Classical conditioning.
2-h. Reciprocal inhibition.
3-g. Operant conditioning.
4-d. Discrimination learning.
5-a. Avoidance learning.

2.9 Learning theory

1-e. Operant conditioning. Trial and error learning (CTP7-413).
2-j. Variable interval reinforcement. This is difficult to extinguish, as rewards are unpredictable.
3-b. Discriminative learning. The behaviour is reinforced only in certain situations.
4-d. Modelling. Learning through observation alone.
5-g. Reciprocal inhibition. One response (anxiety) is inhibited by an opposite response (relaxation).

2.10 Memory

1-i. Semantic memory (Sims-49).
2-d. Recognition (Sims-49).
3-b. Déjà vu (Sims-53).
4-e. Recollection (Sims-49).
5-h. Retrospective falsification (Fish-61).

2.11 Psychological trauma

1-i. Dissolution hypothesis.
2-b. Shattered assumptions.
3-h. Situationally accessible memory.
4-d. Psychological misery.
5-e. Trauma membrane.

3. Psychopathology

3.1 Affective states

Options

a. Affect
b. Affective unresponsiveness
c. Affective blunting
d. Alexithymia
e. Anhedonia
f. Anxiety
g. Elation
h. Euphoria
i. Ecstasy
j. Mood

Lead in

Find one term each for the following descriptions:

Descriptions

1. A state of excessive, unreasonable cheerfulness
2. Lack of emotional sensitivity
3. Fear for no adequate reason
4. Prolonged prevailing feeling states
5. Difficulties in verbalising emotion

3.2 Catatonic symptoms

Options

a. Ambitendency
b. Automatic obedience
c. Catalepsy
d. Cataplexy
e. Co-operation
f. Echopraxia
g. Mitgehen
h. Posturing
i. Stupor
j. Waxy flexibility

Lead in

Identify one term each for the phenomena described below:

Phenomena

1. When the patient was offered a hand to shake, he initially put out his arm to shake hands, then withdrew it, then extended it and repeated this 23 times in rapid succession and his hand finally came to rest without touching the examiner's hand.
2. When the examiner touched the back of patient's forearm with his little finger, his arm moved up. On continued touching, the patient's upper arm stayed at shoulder level and the arm flexed at the elbow.
3. The examiner noticed that patient's muscle tone was uniformly increased. His limbs could be placed in any position. However uncomfortable the position was, he held it for at least ten minutes.
4. The patient's body could be put into any position without any resistance from the patient, although he had been instructed to resist all movements. When the examiner let go of the body part that had been moved, it returned to the resting position.
5. The patient carries out every instruction regardless of the consequences. The examiner asked the patient to put out his tongue and he pricked the patient's tongue with a pin. Every time the examiner asked, the patient obliged and the examiner pricked his tongue.

3.3 Defence mechanisms and disorders

Options

a. Avoidance
b. Displacement
c. Doing and undoing
d. Externalisation
e. Isolation of affect
f. Projection
g. Projective identification
h. Reaction formation
i. Somatisation
j. Splitting

Lead in

Choose the defence mechanisms found in the following disorders:

Disorders

1. Obsessive–compulsive disorder (3)
2. Panic disorder (3)
3. Phobia (3)
4. Post-traumatic stress disorder (2)
5. Paranoid personality disorder (3)

3.4 Delusions

Options

a. Delusion of control
b. Delusion of infidelity
c. Delusion of love
d. Delusion of perception
e. Delusion of reference
f. Delusion of persecution
g. Delusional memory
h. Delusional perception
i. Nihilistic delusion
j. Normal phenomena

Lead in

Find one appropriate term each for the following delusional statements:

Statements

1. "I have no doubt that my wife is having an affair with my neighbour".
2. "They want to control my life, force me to leave my house and to ruin my life".
3. "The television presenter was wearing a purple jacket to indicate that I am gay".
4. "I saw a cat crossing the road and I knew immediately that there is a plot against me".
5. "My intestines are blocked".

3.5 Disorders of perception

Options

a. Autoscopy
b. Command hallucination
c. Delusional perception
d. Functional hallucination
e. Gedankenlautwerden
f. Hyperaesthesia
g. Hypoaesthesia
h. Illusion
i. Pseudohallucination
j. Synaesthesia

Lead in

Select one term each for the following symptoms:

Symptoms

1. When he was walking on a dimly lit street in the night, he felt that he saw figures hiding in the shadows of trees.
2. When a 70-year-old man developed a delirium, his sensory threshold for auditory and pain stimuli were raised and the nurses had to speak loudly to him.
3. A 23-year-old man reported being able to smell music after taking a cocktail of illicit drugs.
4. One week after giving birth, a 33-year-old woman started hearing voices asking her to kill herself and her baby.
5. A 30-year-old man with a diagnosis of schizophrenia complains of hearing his own thoughts aloud.

3.6 First-rank symptoms

Options

a. Delusional perception
b. Passivity of affect
c. Passivity of impulse
d. Running commentary
e. Somatic passivity
f. Third-person auditory hallucinations
g. Thoughts being heard aloud
h. Thought broadcast
i. Thought insertion
j. Thought withdrawal
k. Not a first-rank symptom

Lead in

Find one term each for the phenomena below:

Phenomena

1. "When I heard the stationmaster's whistle, I knew that there was a plot to attack me".
2. "They are using telepathy to make my hands shake".
3. "I do not want to do it, and I don't know who they are, but they are forcing me to do it and I have to try very hard not to do it. This makes me very angry".
4. "When I think hard, I tend to think aloud and my colleagues can hear my thoughts".
5. "They always keep an eye on me. Whatever I am doing, I can hear a male voice reporting to his boss about what I am doing".

3.7 Formal thought disorder

Options

a. Clang association
b. Condensation
c. Derailment
d. Displacement
e. Fusion
f. Flight of ideas
g. Interpenetration
h. Metonyms
i. Overinclusion
j. Substitution

Lead in

Find the appropriate term for the phenomena:

Phenomena

1. Deviation of train of thought without blocking
2. Associations directed by the sound of words rather than their meaning
3. Using one idea for an associated idea
4. Blending two ideas into a false concept
5. Imprecise approximations instead of a more exact word

3.8   Obsessions

Options

a. Compulsion
b. Hoarding
c. Normal phenomenon
d. Not an obsessive–compulsive phenomenon
e. Obsessive drinking
f. Obsessive personality traits
g. Obsessional ritual
h. Obsessional rumination
i. Obsessional slowness
j. Obsessional thoughts

Lead in

Find one term each for the phenomena described below (use one option only once):

Phenomena

1. An office clerk has to cross-check all her work again and again, resulting in her having to work 60 hours, even though her predecessor used to do her job in 20 hours a week.

2. A 40-year-old single woman wants to move from her current house to a bigger one with more storage space, so that she can keep the old issues of the local free newspapers safe.

3. A middle-aged house-proud woman gets up at 6.50 a.m., vacuum cleans her house for 1 hour, reaches work 30 minutes before her office opens, plans out her work weeks in advance and expects her subordinates to be as organised as she is.

4. A young man has recurrent thoughts and mental images of a girl he recently met in a pub. Even though he enjoys these, he wonders why they are so persistent.

5. A 50-year-old man has been working as a chef in a hotel for the past 15 years. He needs to have a glass of wine first thing in the morning and then another one at lunchtime. Once he finishes his shift, he feels a compulsion to drink at least 6 units of alcohol.

3.9   Psychopathology

Options

a. Capgras syndrome
b. Concrete thinking
c. de Clerambault's syndrome
d. Echo de pensee
e. Fregoli delusion
f. Mitmachen
g. Othello syndrome
h. Outcome fear
i. Overvalued idea
j. Tangentiality

Lead in

Select one term each to describe the following phenomena:

Phenomena

1. The patient copies the motor behaviour of the examiner.
2. The patient suffers a panic attack and believes he or she is going to die.
3. The patient believes that another person can radically change their appearance.
4. The patient believes their spouse is unfaithful.
5. The patient answers a question in an indirect and vaguely relevant manner.

3.10 Symptoms

Options

a. Bizarre delusions
b. Hypnopompic hallucinations
c. No persecutory delusions
d. Mood-congruent delusions
e. Preserved psychosocial functioning
f. Prominent affective symptoms
g. Tardive dyskinesia
h. Transient delusions
i. Visual hallucinations
j. Systematised delusions

Lead in

Select two features each that are likely to be present in the conditions below:

Conditions

1. Depression with psychotic features
2. Hypomania
3. Schizophrenia
4. Delusional disorder
5. Delirium

3.11 Thought disorder

Options

a. Asyndesis
b. Condensation
c. Drivelling
d. Faulty use of symbols
e. Fusion
f. Metonyms
g. Neologisms
h. Omission
i. Overinclusion
j. Substitution

Lead in

Find one term each for the following phenomena:

Phenomena

1. A major thought gets substituted by a subsidiary thought
2. Lack of adequate connection between successive thoughts
3. Heterogeneous elements of the thought are interwoven with each other
4. Using the concrete aspects of a symbol instead of its symbolic meaning
5. Senseless omission of a thought or parts of it

Answers

3.1 Affective states

1-h. Euphoria. Usually occurs in organic states, especially frontal lobe disorders (Sims-279; Fish-79).

2-c. Affective blunting (Sims-277; McKenna-24; Fish-74).

3-f. Anxiety (Sims-280; Fish-77).

4-j. Mood is the emotional state prevailing at any given time (Sims-273; McKenna-22; Fish-65).

5-d. Alexithymia (Sims-281).

3.2 Catatonic symptoms

1-a. Ambitendency (Fish-99; Sims-337).

2-g. Mitgehen (Fish-97; Sims-337).

3-j. Waxy flexibility (Fish-101; Sims-336).

4-e. Co-operation (Fish-97).

5-b. Automatic obedience (Sims-337; Fish-94).

3.3 Defence mechanisms and disorders

1-h,c,e. Reaction formation, doing and undoing, isolation of affect (CTP7-601, 1464, CPS7-474).

2-h,i,d. Reaction formation, somatisation, externalisation. Also doing and undoing (CPS7-313).

3-b,a,f. Displacement, avoidance, projection.

4-i,j. Somatisation, splitting. Also minimisation, regression, projective disavowal, dissociation.

5-j,f,g. Splitting, projection, projective identification.

3.4 Delusions

1-b. Delusion of infidelity (CPS7-233).

2-f. Delusion of persecution.

3-e. Delusion of reference.

4-d. Delusional perception.

5-i. Nihilistic delusion.

3.5 Disorders of perception

1-h. Illusion (Fish-15).

2-g. Hypoaesthesia (Fish-15).

3-j. Synaesthesia (Sims-27).

4-b. Command hallucination.

5-e. Gedankenlautwerden (Fish-23).

3.6 First-rank symptoms

1-a. Delusional perception (Sims-107; CPS7-391).
2-e. Somatic passivity (Sims-153; CPS7-391).
3-c. Passivity of impulse (Sims-153; CPS7-391).
4-k. Not a first-rank symptom.
5-d. Running commentary (Sims-151; CPS7-391).

3.7 Formal thought disorder

1-c. Derailment (Fish-50; Sims-149; CPS7-397).
2-a. Clang association.
3-d. Displacement.
4-b. Condensation.
5-h. Metonyms.

3.8 Obsessions

1-i. Obsessional slowness (OTP4-242).
2-b. Hoarding.
3-f. Obsessive personality traits.
4-c. Normal phenomenon. Not unpleasant, not against his will, not irrational.
5-d. Not an obsessive–compulsive phenomenon.

3.9 Psychopathology

1-f. Mitmachen – literally 'make with'.
2-h. Outcome fear – diagnostic of panic disorder.
3-e. Fregoli delusion – named after the French illusionist who could change his appearance.
4-g. Othello syndrome or morbid jealousy.
5-j. Tangentiality.

3.10 Symptoms

1-d,f. Mood-congruent delusions; Prominent affective symptoms (DSM-IV-380).
2-f,c. Prominent affective symptoms; No persecutory delusions (unlike mania) (DSMIV-335).
3-a,j. Bizarre delusions; Systematised delusions (DSM-IV-273).
4-e,j. Preserved psychosocial functioning; Systematized delusions (DSM-IV-296).
5-i,h. Visual hallucinations; Transient delusions (DSM-IV-124).

3.11 Thought disorder

1-j. Substitution (Fish-50).
2-a. Asyndesis (Fish-49; Sims-144).
3-e. Fusion (Fish-50; Sims-140).
4-d. Faulty use of symbols (Fish-49).
5-h. Omission (Fish-50).

4. Neurosciences

4.1   Agnosias and apraxias

Options

a. Agraphognosia
b. Anosognosia
c. Astereognosia
d. Constructional apraxia
e. Dressing apraxia
f. Hemisomatognosis
g. Ideomotor apraxia
h. Prosopagnosia
i. Simultagnosia
j. Visual agnosia

Lead in

Select one term each for the following presentations:

Presentations

1. An inability to recognise faces
2. An inability to carry out a requested movement properly
3. A failure to recognise the whole of a complex picture while being able to identify individual parts
4. The feeling that the limbs on one side of the body are missing
5. An inability to copy a complex pattern

4.2   Eye signs

Options

a. Argyll Robertson pupils
b. Holmes–Adie pupil
c. Horner's syndrome
d. Hutchinson pupil
e. Mid-brain lesion
f. Miotic drugs
g. Mydriatic drugs
h. Oculomotor nerve lesion
i. Pontine lesion
j. Senile pupils

Lead in

Match one cause each for the following clinical pictures:

Clinical pictures

1. Ptosis, enophthalmos and anhydrosis with normal light and accommodation reflex
2. Irregular pupils with absent light reflex and normal accommodation reflex
3. Ptosis, eye turned 'downwards and outwards' with absent light and accommodation reflex
4. Sluggish light and accommodation reflexes
5. Pupil on one side constricts and then widely dilates. Then the other pupil goes through the same sequence

4.3 Functional neuroanatomy

Options

a. Amygdala
b. Cerebellar vermis
c. Fusiform gyrus
d. Left inferior frontal cortex
e. Medulla oblongata
f. Nucleus accumbens
g. Optic radiation
h. Posterior superior temporal lobe
i. Pons
j. Superior parietal cortex

Lead in

Identify one area each that is most important in the following functions:

Functions

1. Recognition of faces
2. Reward processing
3. Generation of speech
4. Fear
5. Comprehension of language

4.4   Glial cells

Options

a. Apoptosis
b. Information processing
c. Lining the wall of the ventricular system
d. Long-term potentiation
e. Myelination of axons in the peripheral nervous system
f. Myelination of axons in the central nervous system
g. Phagocytosis
h. Regulation of circadian rhythms
i. Removal or degradation neurotransmitters released into the interstitial space
j. Storage of neurotransmitters

Lead in

Identify one function each of the following glial cells:

Glial cells

1. Microglia
2. Astrocytes
3. Ependymal cells
4. Oligodendrocytes
5. Schwann cells

4.5 Neuroanatomical localisation

Options

a. Attention
b. Calculation
c. Complex visuo-perceptual skills
d. Constructional abilities
e. Language
f. Memory
g. Personality
h. Praxis
i. Prosody

Lead in

Identify three functions each with the following localisations:

Localisations

1. Localised in the non-dominant hemisphere
2. Localised in the dominant hemisphere
3. Distributed functions, not strictly lateralised

4.6   Neuroanatomical regions

Options

a. Prefrontal cortext
b. Basal ganglia
c. Cerebellum
d. Diencephalon
e. Medulla oblongata
f. Metencephalon
g. Midbrain
h. Occipital lobe
i. Parietal lobe
j. Pons
k. Temporal lobe

Lead in

Match one brain region each with the following structures:

Structures

1. Ventral tegmental area
2. Area V1
3. Striatum
4. Entorhinal cortex
5. Hypothalamus

4.7   Neuropathology of dementias

Options

a. Adrenoleucodystrophy
b. Alzheimer's disease
c. Frontotemporal dementia
d. Huntington's disease
e. Lewy body dementia
f. Multiple sclerosis
g. Normal pressure hydrocephalus
h. Pick's disease
i. Shy–Drager syndrome
j. Vascular dementia

Lead in

Choose one condition that best fits the descriptions below. Each option may be used more than once:

Descriptions

1. Neuritic plaques are almost universal
2. Neurofibrillary tangles are present and usually considered essential for diagnosis
3. Numerous rounded inclusion bodies within the neurons
4. Cystic formation with lacunar changes and reactive gliosis
5. Balloon cells and Hirano bodies

4.8 Pathophysiology

Options

a. Beta-amyloid precursor protein
b. Dorsal raphe nucleus serotonin
c. Glutamate-induced neuronal calcium influx
d. Hippocampal cholinergic
e. Mammillary body alpha-ketoglutarate
f. Prions
g. Subcortical leukomalacia
h. Tau protein
i. Tuberoinfundibular dopaminergic
j. Ventral tegmental area dopamine/enkephalin

Lead in

Match the following conditions with one pathophysiological mechanism each:

Conditions

1. Korsakoff's psychosis
2. Corticobasal degeneration
3. Binswanger's disease
4. Alcoholic reward mechanism
5. Alzheimer's disease

4.9   Pathophysiology of schizophrenia

Options

a. Broca's area
b. Cerebellum
c. Hippocampus
d. Lateral ventricles
e. Left inferior frontal cortex
f. Mammillary bodies
g. Medulla oblongata
h. Occipital cortex
i. Pons
j. Prefrontal cortex
k. Red nucleus
l. Striatum

Lead in

With regard to schizophrenia, match each pathological/
pathophysiological finding with one neuro-anatomical area:

Findings

1. Excess dopamine release here on amphetamine challenge
2. D_2 occupancy here, by haloperidol, predicts antipsychotic response, drug-induced extrapyramidal side effects, akathisia, and prolactin elevation
3. Neuroimaging studies suggest decreased activity here
4. Increased volume
5. A disproportionate decrease in volume

Answers

4.1 Agnosias and apraxias

1-h. Prosopagnosia (Lishman-22).
2-g. Ideomotor apraxia.
3-i. Simultagnosia.
4-f. Hemisomatognosis.
5-d. Constructional apraxia.

4.2 Eye signs

1-c. Horner's syndrome (NFP-25).
2-a. Argyll Robertson pupils. Occurs in diabetes mellitus and neurosyphilis. The iris shows patchy atrophy and depigmentation (OM4-56; NFP-26).
3-h. Oculomotor nerve lesion (NFP-25).
4-b. Holmes–Adie pupil. A benign condition. Usually occurs in women. Unilateral in 80% of cases. Associated with diminished ankle and knee reflexes (OM4-56).
5-d. Hutchinson pupil. This refers to the sequence of events resulting from rapidly rising unilateral intracranial pressure, e.g. in intracranial haemorrhage (OM4-56).

4.3 Functional neuroanatomy

1-c. Fusiform gyrus.
2-f. Nucleus accumbens (PNS-1009).
3-d. Left inferior frontal cortex (Broca's area) (Hodges-48).
4-a. Amygdala (PNS-988).
5-h. Posterior superior temporal lobe (Wernicke's area) (Hodges-48).

4.4 Glial cells

1-g. Phagocytosis (CTP7-4).
2-i. Removal or degradation neurotransmitters released into the interstitial space.
3-c. Lining the wall of the ventricular system.
4-f. Myelination of axons in the central nervous system.
5-e. Myelination of axons in the peripheral nervous system.

4.5 Neuroanatomical localisation

1-c,d,i.   Complex visuo-perceptual skills, constructional abilities, prosody (Hodges-44).
2-e,b,h.   Language, calculation, praxis.
3-f,a,g.   Memory, attention, personality.

4.6 Neuroanatomical regions

1-g.   Midbrain (Fitzgerald & Folan-Curran).
2-h.   Occipital lobe.
3-b.   Basal ganglia.
4-k.   Temporal lobe.
5-d.   Diencephalon.

4.7 Neuropathology of dementias

1-b.   Alzheimer's disease (Lishman-428).
2-b.   Alzheimer's disease.
3-e.   Lewy body dementia.
4-j.   Vascular dementia.
5-h.   Pick's disease.

4.8 Pathophysiology

1-e.   Mammillary body alpha-ketoglutarate.
2-h.   Tau protein.
3-g.   Subcortical leukomalacia.
4-j.   Ventral tegmental area dopamine/enkephalin.
5-a.   Beta-amyloid precursor protein.

4.9 Pathophysiology of schizophrenia

1-l.   Striatum. Suggests pre-synaptic dopamine receptor abnormalities (OTP4-606).
2-l.   Striatum (Kapur et al, 2000).
3-j.   Prefrontal cortex (OTP4-607).
4-d.   Lateral ventricles (OTP4-608).
5-c.   Hippocampus (OTP4-608).

5. Assessment and classification

5.1 Aetiological factors

Options

a. Alcohol
b. Being involved in an accident 2 months ago
c. Childhood sexual abuse
d. HIV positive
e. Impaired hearing
f. Perinatal hypoxia
g. Reduced visual acuity
h. Regular use of non-steroidal anti-inflammatory drugs (NSAIDs)
i. Smoking
j. Use of corticosteroids

Lead in

Select one risk factor each associated with the following clinical situations:

Clinical situations

1. A young man with mood-incongruent auditory hallucinations, complex delusions and social withdrawal.
2. A 26-year-old male with low moods, recurrent nightmares, flashbacks and avoidance.
3. A 45-year-old male with encephalopathy, confusion, ataxia and ophthalmoplegia.
4. A cognitively intact older man with visual hallucinations.
5. A 33-year-old female with affective instability, intense emotions and relationships, and frequent wrist cutting.

5.2 Aetiology

Options

a. Alcohol
b. Being an oldest child
c. Childhood sexual abuse
d. Diabetes
e. HLA DR15-DQ6
f. Impaired hearing
g. Loss of mother before age 14 years
h. Being a migrant
i. Reduced visual acuity
j. Regular use of NSAIDs
k. Smoking

Lead in

Select one risk factor each that is strongly associated with the following clinical situations:

Clinical situations

1. A young man with mood-incongruent complex delusions and social withdrawal
2. A young woman with disrupted sleep, low self-esteem, and weight loss
3. A 75-year old woman living alone with first onset of both somatic and auditory hallucinations and persecutory delusions
4. Anterograde amnesia
5. Repeated acute episodes of collapse precipitated by laughing

5.3   Aetiology of dementias

Options

a. Adrenoleucodystrophy
b. Creutzfeldt–Jakob disease (CJD)
c. Ganser's syndrome
d. Gerstmann's syndrome
e. Gerstmann–Straussler syndrome
f. Koro
g. Kuru
h. Multiple sclerosis
i. Normal pressure hydrocephalus
j. Progressive multifocal leucoencephalopathy

Lead in

Choose one option each that best corresponds to the statements below:

Statements

1. Subacute brain degeneration caused by a transmissible agent leading to dementia; this is restricted to New Guinea
2. Clinically and pathologically similar to CJD but with a longer duration to death
3. It can complicate acquired immune deficiency syndrome (AIDS) or disorders of the reticuloendothelial system
4. This is probably the best known of the human spongiform encephalopathies and consists essentially of a dementing illness that runs a very rapid course
5. Development of memory impairment over weeks to months, unsteady gait and urinary incontinence

5.4 Classification

Options

a. Absence seizures
b. Alcohol intoxication
c. Global assessment of functioning = 70
d. Major depressive disorder, single episode, in full remission
e. Mild mental retardation
f. Narcolepsy
g. No diagnosis/none
h. Obsessive–compulsive personality features
i. Psychotic disorder due a general medical condition
j. Unemployment

Lead in

Group the above options into the following axes on DSM-IV (each option may fit into one or more axes):

Axes

1. Axis I (5)
2. Axis II (3)
3. Axis III (2)
4. Axis IV (2)
5. Axis V (1)

5.5 Interview

Options

a. Clarification
b. Closed questioning
c. Confrontation
d. Empathy
e. Eliciting precision
f. Facilitation
g. Interpretation
h. Reflection
i. Summarising
j. Sympathy

Lead in

Select one technique each that is used in the following statements:

Statements

1. "What do you mean when you say you have been having panic attacks?"
2. "Before we talk about the panic attacks can I just go through what you have told me about your depression? Please correct me as I go along".
3. "I can see that things have been very tough for you recently".
4. "Go on . . . Tell me more about it".
5. "You seem quite upset when you are talking about this".

5.6   Interview techniques

Options

a. Adhering
b. Confrontation
c. Encouragement
d. Facilitation
e. Legitimation
f. Negotiating
g. Offering hope
h. Reassurance
i. Respectful statements
j. Support

Lead in

Name the technique used in these statements:

Statements

1. "I want to offer what help that I can".
2. "I think there are ways that we can work together to help you feel better".
3. "You have managed before and you can do it again".
4. "I am impressed by what you have managed to do despite all this".
5. "It is quite acceptable to feel the way you do".

5.7   Physical findings

Options

a. Amygdala atrophy
b. Cerebral oedema
c. Ebstein's anomaly
d. Hepatic transaminase elevation
e. Hyperprolactinaemia
f. Impaired glucose tolerance
g. Maldevelopment of the cerebellum
h. Reduced hippocampal volumes
i. Sick euthyroid syndrome
j. Retinitis pigmentosa

Lead in

Match one physical finding with each of the following disorders/
treatments:

Disorders/treatments

1. Lithium therapy
2. PTSD
3. Autism
4. Olanzapine therapy
5. Anorexia nervosa

5.8   Risk of schizophrenia

Options

a. 1
b. 5
c. 10
d. 30
e. 50
f. 75
g. Greater
h. Reduced
i. Similar
j. The same

Lead in

Select one option each for the following statements. Each option may be used more than once:

Statements

1. In first-episode schizophrenia, comparing longer versus shorter durations of untreated psychosis, the response to treatment is ___ with longer durations.
2. Comparing children at high risk of schizophrenia with controls, IQ is ___ in high-risk children.
3. The risk of schizophrenia is ___ % if one parent has schizophrenia.
4. The risk of schizophrenia is ___ % if both parents have schizophrenia.
5. Comparing high-risk individuals with schizophrenic first-degree versus second-degree relatives, ventricular volume is ___ in the first-degree group.

Answers

5.1 Aetiological factors

1-f. Perinatal hypoxia – a risk factor for schizophrenia (OTP4-347).
2-b. Being involved in an accident 2 months ago. A criterion for PTSD.
3-a. Alcohol. Wernicke–Korsakoff's syndrome.
4-g. Reduced visual acuity. A risk factor for visual hallucination in the elderly.
5-c. Childhood sexual abuse. A risk factor for borderline personality disorder (OTP4-177).

5.2 Aetiology

1-h. Being a migrant. Migrants have a higher risk for psychosis, e.g. Norwegian migrants to the USA (Ødegärd, 1932), people of African-Caribbean origin in the UK, children born in Greenland to Danish mothers (Mortensen et al, 1999).
2-g. Loss of mother before age 14 – a risk factor for depression (Brown & Harris).
3-f. Impaired hearing – a risk factor for late-onset psychosis.
4-a. Alcohol. Alcoholic Korsakoff's syndrome is characterised by anterograde amnesia.
5-e. HLA DR15-DQ6. Cataplexy is a symptom of narcolepsy. Narcolepsy has a strong association with HLA type.

5.3 Aetiology of dementias

1-g. Kuru (Lishman-688).
2-e. Gerstmann–Straussler syndrome.
3-j. Progressive multifocal leucoencephalopathy.
4-b. Creutzfeldt–Jakob disease.
5-i. Normal pressure hydrocephalus.

5.4 Classification

1-b,d,f,g,i. Alcohol intoxication, major depressive disorder, narcolepsy, no diagnosis, psychotic disorder due to a general medical condition (DSM-IV-25).
2-e,g,h. Mild mental retardation, no diagnosis, obsessive–compulsive personality features.
3-a,g. Absence seizures, no diagnosis.
4-g,j. None, unemployment.
5-c. Global assessment of functioning = 70.

5.5 Interview

1-a. Clarification (CPS7-221).
2-i. Summarising.
3-d. Empathy – the ability to reflect accurately the inner experience of another person.
4-f. Facilitation.
5-h. Reflection – stating or labelling the observed emotion.

5.6 Interview techniques

1-j. Support, indicating and emphasising the interviewer's role in helping.
2-g. Offering hope, that a problem can be resolved.
3-c. Encouragement.
4-i. Respectful statements, which positively reinforce the person's ability to cope.
5-e. Legitimation, indicating not only that it is OK to talk about these feelings but that it is quite acceptable for the person to feel the way he does.

5.7 Physical findings

1-c. Ebstein's anomaly.
2-h. Reduced hippocampal volumes.
3-g. Maldevelopment of the cerebellum.
4-f. Impaired glucose tolerance.
5-i. Sick euthyroid syndrome.

5.8 Risk of schizophrenia

1-h. Reduced (Ucok *et al*, 2004).
2-h. Reduced (Niemi *et al*, 2003).
3-c. 10.
4-e. 50.
5-g. Greater.

6. Clinical syndromes

6.1   Alcohol and drugs

Options

a. Acute intoxication due to use of alcohol
b. Alcohol–disulfiram interaction
c. Alcoholic memory blackout
d. Alcoholic hallucinosis
e. Amnesic syndrome
f. Delirium tremens
g. Extradural haemorrhage
h. Pathological intoxication
i. Schizophrenia
j. Status epilepticus

Lead in

His girlfriend drags a 36-year-old man to the A&E department. They are poor historians and they change their stories often. Match each scenario with one diagnosis:

Scenarios

1. The girlfriend says that he got drunk and fell off the staircase. He had worsening headache, vomiting and fits. On examination, he has disorientation, brisk reflexes, upgoing plantar, hemiparesis and bleeding from his ears.
2. The girlfriend says that he stopped drinking 3 days ago. Since last night he has been frightened, sweating, shaky, not sleeping and trying to catch imaginary mice running across the room.
3. The girlfriend says that he stopped drinking 4 months ago. However he started hearing threatening voices. She feels that he was better off drinking than not drinking and being threatened by these voices.
4. The girlfriend says that in the previous night, he got drunk, but behaved well and walked back home. This morning he could not remember anything about the previous night.
5. He complains of a throbbing headache, palpitations, nausea and vomiting. He is hypotensive and has facial flushing. He says that the medication that was meant to stop his drinking is not working.

6.2 Anorexia

Options

a. Bradycardia with hypotension
b. Decreased
c. High T3 and low growth hormone
d. Low T3 and high growth hormone
e. Metabolic acidosis
f. Metabolic alkalosis
g. Microcytic hypochromic anaemia with thrombocytosis
h. Normocytic normochromic anaemia with thrombocytopenia
i. Raised
j. Tachycardia with hypertension

Lead in

Choose one option each for the following complications in anorexia nervosa:

Complications

1. Cardiovascular complications
2. Electrolyte abnormality caused by laxative abuse
3. Endocrine abnormalities
4. The levels of cholesterol and free fatty acids are ____
5. Haematological complications

6.3   Anxiety disorders

Options

a. Acute stress reaction
b. Adjustment disorder
c. Agoraphobia
d. Generalised anxiety disorder
e. Mixed anxiety and depressive disorder
f. Panic disorder, moderate
g. Panic disorder, severe
h. PTSD
i. Social phobia
j. Specific phobia

Lead in

Select one diagnosis each for the following scenarios:

Scenarios

1. A 23-year-old woman presents with complaints of repeated, discrete episodes of palpitations, breathlessness, dizziness and fear of dying. No physical cause has been found. These episodes occur 4–5 times per month and are not related to any particular situation.

2. A 30-year-old man describes himself as a life-long worrier. His worrying has worsened in the past 6 months following his being made redundant. His worries keep him awake in the night. He has chest pains, muscle aches and difficulty taking a full deep breath.

3. A man brings his 49-year-old wife to the A&E department. She is dazed, confused, disorientated, agitated and is restlessly pacing. She was well until this morning, when she heard about her only son being admitted to an intensive care unit in a critical state following a road traffic accident.

4. A 20-year-old man has returned home from the university. He feels very anxious about presenting his projects. He is worried that his teachers and colleagues will ridicule him. He also admits to taking alcohol at times to overcome this fear.

5. A 45-year-old woman refuses to leave home because she becomes very anxious when she is away from home, travelling in buses or when she is in the town. She only goes out if she is with a family member.

6.4 Bereavement

Options

a. Adjustment reaction
b. Anniversary reaction
c. Anticipatory grief
d. Delayed grief
e. Distorted grief
f. Prolonged grief
g. Severe depressive episode
h. Stage one of bereavement
i. Stage two of bereavement
j. Stage three of bereavement

Lead in

Choose one term each for the following scenarios:

Scenarios

1. Her husband brought a young mother to the A&E department after she took a large overdose of painkillers. She has been devastated by the death of her child 3 months ago. She feels that she deserves to die. She feels guilty and blames herself for another baby's death on the TV. She spends all day in bed.
2. One month after the death of her sister, a woman visits her GP for help. She is pining for her sister and still very tearful. She can't sleep and has a poor appetite. Recently she has been comforted by the voice of her late sister and she feels her presence late at night.
3. A 70-year-old woman was very dependent on her husband, who died suddenly of a heart attack 3 weeks previously. She has no other family. Her neighbour is concerned that she does not seem bothered; she has not cried and is carrying on as before.
4. Whilst attending the family Christmas, a 28-year-old man became acutely distressed and agitated on seeing his late brother's photo on the mantelpiece. It was 3 years since his brother's death. He yelled at his parents and blamed them for his brother's death. He couldn't sleep that night and had flashbacks of the funeral.
5. Fifteen months after the death of his wife, a 55-year-old man had only managed to return to work part time. He feels lonely in the evenings but cannot face mixing with people. He has difficulty falling asleep. He can't be bothered to cook for himself and lives off microwave meals. He does not see any purpose in life, but has no plans of suicide.

6.5 Clinical diagnoses

Options

a. Adjustment disorder
b. Bipolar illness
c. Depressive episode
d. Emotionally unstable personality disorder – borderline type
e. Emotionally unstable personality disorder – impulsive type
f. Generalised anxiety disorder
g. Hypochondriasis
h. PTSD
i. Schizophrenia
j. Somatisation disorder

Lead in

Select one diagnosis each for the following presentations:

Presentations

1. A 40-year-old woman has visited her GP surgery twice a month for 5 years, rotating through all the GPs in the practice. She has complained at various times of bloating, diarrhoea, irregular and painful periods, aches and pains in her abdomen, head, chest and joints, insomnia, fatigue, and numbness and tingling of her hands. She can't be reassured.
2. A 40-year-old lawyer has been concerned that the sensation of his heartbeat has altered. He has been to his GP, a local cardiologist and a Harley Street cardiologist and had numerous examinations and extensive investigations, all of which were normal. However, his problems continue. He has stopped working. He spends long hours on the Internet seeking information on heart problems. He is convinced that something has been missed. He is seeking another specialist opinion.
3. A 19-year-old college student presented with persecutory ideas, sadness, distress, lack of concentration and perplexity. He also complained of lack of interest and loss of appetite. His academic performance has deteriorated recently. There was no evidence of hallucinations or thought interference.
4. A 34-year-old man presents with a three-month history of exhaustion and weight loss. He has no interest in anything and has no motivation.
5. A 29-year-old woman was arrested for assaulting her boyfriend of 3 weeks' standing. He accused her of seeing people only as either very good or very bad, telling different things to his different friends and accusing him of trying to abandon her. She complained of chronic low mood and feelings of boredom. She has a long history of self-harm episodes. She was sexually abused between the ages of 7 and 11 years by her mother's boyfriend.

6.6 Clinical features

Options

a. Anorexia nervosa
b. Binge eating disorder
c. Body dysmorphic disorder
d. Bulimia nervosa
e. Diogenes syndrome
f. Mania with psychotic symptoms
g. Morbid obesity
h. Psychotic depression
i. Pica
j. Temporal lobe epilepsy

Lead in

Match each clinical feature with one option:

Clinical features

1. Bradycardia
2. Lead poisoning
3. Vital exhaustion
4. Overvalued idea that buttocks are misshapen
5. A large collection of rotten foodstuffs

6.7 Clinical features of anxiety disorders

Options

a. Acute stress reaction
b. Adjustment disorder – brief depressive reaction
c. Agoraphobia with panic disorder
d. Claustrophobia
e. Depressive episode
f. Generalised anxiety disorder
g. Mixed anxiety and depressive disorder
h. Panic disorder
i. PTSD
j. Social phobia

Lead in

Find one diagnosis each that best fits the following scenarios:

Scenarios

1. A 35-year-old woman is frightened to leave her flat. She feels anxious travelling on the bus and shopping at the supermarket. Whenever she goes shopping alone she has a panic attack and has to run out of the shop. Hence, her sister helps her with the weekly shopping.
2. An 18-year-old boy was sent home from school because he was drunk just before he was due to give a presentation. He is spending more time alone. His friends have stopped calling as he seldom goes out with them anymore. He is refusing to go out for a family meal for his father's birthday as he says he would be so tense he may vomit.
3. A 30-year-old man was involved in a car crash when his co-passenger was badly injured. He now drives the longer way to work to avoid travelling down the same road. He has insomnia and nightmares. He feels constantly wound up and argues a lot with his wife.
4. A 42-year-old woman attended A&E following a small overdose of her sleeping pills. She wanted her husband to take more notice of her. Since he asked her for a divorce a week ago she is not coping and constantly worries about the future. Work is a distraction for her and she still enjoys going out with friends to take her mind off things.
5. A 64-year-old woman has been to A&E twice in the last month with suspected heart attack, but her ECGs were normal. She complains of episodes of chest pain, palpitations and difficulty catching her breath. This comes on suddenly out of the blue and lasts up to 10 minutes. During these episodes she feels she is going to die.

6.8   Clinical pictures

Options

a. Allodynia
b. Approximate answers
c. Chronic fatigue
d. Cognitive impairment
e. Dyspareunia
f. Hysterical blindness
g. Memory loss
h. Non-cardiac chest pain
i. Secondary gain
j. Somatosensory amplification

Lead in

Match each of the following conditions with its one most characteristic feature:

Conditions

1. Persistent somatoform pain disorder
2. Somatisation
3. Conversion disorder
4. Panic disorder
5. Briquet's disorder

6.9 Clinical syndromes

Options

a. Adjustment disorder with anxiety
b. Borderline personality disorder
c. Cyclothymic disorder
d. Fronto-temporal dementia
e. HIV encephalopathy
f. PTSD
g. Rapid-cycling bipolar disorder
h. Schizophreniform psychosis
i. Bipolar II disorder
j. Paranoid personality disorder

Lead in

Match the clinical scenarios with one diagnosis each:

Clinical scenarios

1. A 29-year-old intravenous drug user displaying fatuous mood and slowed cognition
2. An 82-year-old former serviceman with irritability and avoidant behaviour following a road traffic accident
3. A 31-year-old man on lithium for bipolar affective disorder was started on venlafaxine 7 months ago. Since then, he had one episode each of depression, mixed affective state and mania and two episodes of hypomania
4. A 42-year-old schoolteacher with non-cardiac chest pain following a complaint made by a student
5. A 31-year-old homosexual man experiences euphoria, increased libido and decreased need for sleep 2 days after commencing venlafaxine

6.10 Complications of anorexia

Options

a. Hypercortisolaemia
b. Hypophosphataemia
c. Hypofolataemia
d. Hypoglycaemia
e. Hypokalaemia
f. Hyponatraemia
g. Hypothiaminaemia
h. Hypothyroidism
i. Hypo-oestrogenaemia
j. Osteoporosis

Lead in

Match one pathophysiological cause each for the physical complications of anorexia nervosa:

Complications

1. Sudden death during refeeding
2. Respiratory failure
3. Disturbed lower limb proprioception
4. Muscle weakness in purging-type anorexia
5. Coma during fluid resuscitation

6.11 Culture-bound syndromes

Options

a. Amok
b. Ataque de Nervios
c. Brain Fag
d. Dhat
e. Koro
f. Latah
g. Pibloktoq
h. Susto
i. Taijin Kyofusho
j. Windigo

Lead in

Identify the following clinical scenarios:

Scenarios

1. A 24-year-old Indonesian woman presents with a highly exaggerated response to a fright in a trance-like state with echopraxia, echolalia and command obedience.

2. A 27-year-old Chinese gentleman presents with an acute panic attack and intense fear that his penis is shrinking into his abdomen. He anticipates that this will ultimately cause his death.

3. A 32-year-old Eskimo woman presents with an abrupt dissociative episode lasting 1 hour. This is characterised by extreme agitation including tearing off her clothes and rolling in the snow. This is followed by collapse and complete amnesia for the episode.

4. A 22-year-old native of North America presents with depression, suicidal thoughts and a delusional compulsion to eat human flesh.

5. An 18-year-old west African student preparing for exams presents in a state of distress with inability to concentrate, poor memory and pains in his head and neck.

6.12 Diagnosis of anxiety disorders

Options

a. Acute stress reaction
b. Agoraphobia
c. Depressive episode with anxiety symptoms
d. Generalised anxiety disorder
e. Mixed anxiety and depressive disorder
f. Phobic disorder
g. PTSD
h. Social phobia
i. Conversion disorder
j. Somatisation disorder

Lead in

Find one diagnosis each for the following conditions:

Conditions

1. A 35-year-old male presents with a lifelong pattern of worrying. Of late, his anxiety has been increasing and interfering with his work and social life. There are no precipitating factors and he feels anxious and 'on the edge' all the time.

2. A 32-year-old woman has an intense fear of going out. When she has to go out, she usually cannot sleep the night before and worries excessively. She fears being alone and in situations that she cannot escape from.

3. A 28-year-old male has a fear of meeting people. He feels that others are scrutinising him and that he will do something embarrassing or humiliating.

4. A 26-year-old firefighter presents with low moods 4 months after he witnessed a fire in which a three-year-old child was burnt to death. He reports nightmares, intrusive thoughts and flashbacks about the incident. He has stopped going to work.

5. A 25-year-old single mother, who was made redundant a week ago, presents with sudden onset of paralysis of the right hand and convulsions. Physical examinations and extensive investigations carried out were negative. She is seemingly unconcerned about her symptoms.

6.13 Diagnosis of eating disorders

Options

a. Addison's disease
b. Anorexia nervosa
c. Bulimia nervosa
d. Coeliac disease
e. Cushing's disease
f. Endometriosis
g. Hyperthyroidism
h. Irritable bowel syndrome
i. Systemic lupus erythematosus
j. Tuberculosis

Lead in

Choose one diagnosis each for the following scenarios:

Scenarios

1. The parents of a 14-year-old girl are concerned about her low weight and her having not attained menarche. She believes that she has to go a long way in achieving her ideal weight and avoids fatty foods. Her body mass index (BMI) was 16.5.
2. The domineering parents of Di, a 24-year-old female are concerned about her weight loss and infrequent menstrual periods. The mother feels that the father's critical attitude causes Di's tremors and frequent stools. Di refuses to put the central heating on in her flat because it makes her sweat. The father thinks that Di is deliberately trying to keep the nagging mother away.
3. A 35-year-old woman is concerned about hyperpigmentation in her buccal mucosa. She is pleased about her recent weight loss. On questioning she reported nausea, constipation, abdominal pains, joint and muscle pains, and feeling dizzy and being confused at times.
4. A 25-year-old female complains of being too fat and feeling low. She tries to 'diet' by making herself sick and by using laxatives. However she often loses control and eats huge amounts of food over short periods of time then feels guilty and makes herself sick. Her body weight is normal.
5. A 50-year-old woman presents to her GP with complaints of weight loss. She also has bulky, foul-smelling stools, abdominal pain, bloating, nausea, vomiting, angular stomatitis and ulcers in her mouth. The gastroenterologist found villous atrophy on jejunal biopsy.

6.14 Dissociative disorders

Options

a. Conversion disorder

b. Dissociative amnesia

c. Fugue

d. Ganser's syndrome

e. Multiple personality disorder

f. Munchausen syndrome by proxy

g. Munchausen syndrome

h. Possession disorder

i. Retrograde amnesia

j. Somatisation

Lead in

Find one most appropriate term for each of the following scenarios:

Scenarios

1. A 42-year-old male was found roaming the streets of London. He spoke with a northern accent. He did not know where he was or had been over the past few days.

2. A policeman who works in town A was found in town B, 100 miles away, where he was known for his antisocial behaviour. When questioned, he was not aware that he was a policeman.

3. A 33-year-old ex-nurse repeatedly presents to the A&E department with multiple complaints. She had multiple explorative surgeries and no pathology has been found. When admitted with generalised infection, at a psychiatric consultation, she admitted to injecting faeces into her body.

4. A 43-year-old male was involved in a car accident 3 days previously and sustained a head injury. Now he is unable to recall anything that happened in the 2 days prior to the accident.

5. A 28-year-old single mother repeatedly brings her two-year-old child to the hospital. He has been extensively investigated. This time she has presented with complaints that the child has haematuria. An extensive workup showed no cause.

6.15 Drug intoxication and withdrawal

Options

a. Dysphoric mood
b. Inco-ordination
c. Increased appetite
d. Nausea
e. Nystagmus
f. Pupillary dilatation
g. Seizures
h. Slurred speech
i. Vivid dreams
j. Yawning

Lead in

Choose three features for each condition:

Conditions

1. Amphetamine intoxication
2. Cocaine withdrawal
3. Inhalant intoxication
4. Opiate withdrawal
5. Benzodiazepine intoxication

6.16 Epidemiology of suicide

Options

a. 50 times
b. 100 times
c. 40%
d. 66%
e. 3:1
f. 6:1
g. Depressive disorders
h. Personality disorders
i. Social classes I and V
j. Social classes II, III and IV

Lead in

Match one option each with the demographics related to suicide:

Demographics

1. The ratio of men:women committing suicide in the UK
2. Higher rates are found among these social classes
3. The commonest psychiatric disorder in those committing suicide
4. The rate of suicide in the year following deliberate self-harm is raised by
5. The percentage of people who see their GP in the month prior to committing suicide

6.17 Late-onset schizophrenia

Options

a. Approximately 25%
b. Earlier
c. Higher
d. Later
e. Less impaired
f. Less than 10%
g. Lower
h. Men
i. More impaired
j. Women

Lead in

Match one option each with the following statements:

Statements

1. The proportion of patients with schizophrenia whose illness first emerges after the age of 40 has been estimated to be ___
2. Onset of schizophrenia among women is ___ than in men.
3. In late-onset cases there is over-representation among ___.
4. The risk for schizophrenia in relatives of patients with very late-onset schizophrenia is ___ compared to those with schizophrenia of early onset.
5. In late-onset as compared with early-onset schizophrenia, premorbid educational, occupational and psychosocial functioning is ___.

6.18 Paraphilias

Options

a. Dual-role transvestism
b. Exhibitionism
c. Fetishism
d. Fetishistic transvestism
e. Frotteurism
f. Pedophilia
g. Sadomasochism
h. Sexual sadism
i. Transsexualism
j. Voyeurism

Lead in

Choose one term each for the following scenarios:

Scenarios

1. A 40-year-old single man wants to be referred for a sex change surgery. He says that he feels like a woman and would like to change his body and his way of living in order to be accepted as a woman.

2. A 35-year-old man was brought to his GP by a friend who is concerned that he wears women's clothes at home and outside. He seems amused and denies wanting to change his sex or having any sexual arousal on wearing the clothes. He claims that he just wants to experience a temporary membership of the opposite sex.

3. A 45-year-old married man's wife is concerned about him wearing her undergarments and shoes. He claims that dressing this way makes him feel sexually satisfied and he does so to get the feeling of being a woman.

4. A 50-year-old man was arrested for exposing his genitals to women on the street. He did not know these women. He has not approached them in any other way. He has had no previous convictions.

5. A 20-year-old man was arrested following complaints from a women's hostel warden that he has been peeping into their bathrooms.

6.19 Personality disorders

Options

a. Antisocial
b. Avoidant
c. Borderline personality disorder
d. Dependent
e. Histrionic
f. Mixed personality disorder
g. Narcissistic
h. Obsessive–compulsive
i. Paranoid
j. Schizoid

Lead in

Choose the personality disorders that fit with the following criteria:

Criteria

1. Cluster A Personality disorder (2)
2. Cluster B Personality disorder (4)
3. Cluster C Personality disorder (2)
4. These specific terms not used in ICD-10 (5)
5. These specific terms not used in DSM4 (1)

6.20 Personality traits

Options

a. Allusive thinking
b. Emotionally aloof
c. Failure to plan ahead
d. Feelings of emptiness and boredom
e. Grandiose
f. Haughty and entitled
g. Impressionistic speech
h. Parsimony
i. Preference for solitary activities
j. Suspiciousness

Lead in

Match one personality trait each with the personality disorders:

Personality disorders

1. Schizotypal
2. Antisocial
3. Obsessive–compulsive
4. Histrionic
5. Borderline

6.21 Sexual dysfunction

Options

a. Diabetes mellitus
b. Fluoxetine
c. Papaverine
d. Performance anxiety
e. Phenylephrine
f. Sensate focus techniques and graduated masturbation
g. Sensate focus techniques and graduated vaginal dilatation
h. Squeeze technique
i. Traumatic early sexual experience
j. Trazodone

Lead in

Choose one cause and one treatment for each condition (use each option only once):

Conditions

1. Premature ejaculation
2. Vaginismus
3. Erectile impotence
4. Priapism
5. Anorgasmia

6.22 Somatoform disorders

Options

a. Body dysmorphic disorder
b. Depersonalisation disorder
c. Dissociative fugue state
d. Ganser's syndrome
e. Hypochondriacal disorder
f. Multiple personality disorder
g. Munchausen syndrome
h. Possession disorder
i. Somatisation disorder
j. Somatoform pain disorder

Lead in

Find one term each for the following scenarios:

Scenarios

1. A 53-year-old woman has been complaining of abdominal pain and bloating accompanied by shortness of breath, chest pain and a tingling sensation of limbs that has been present for the past 2 years. No physical cause has been found despite extensive investigations.
2. A 40-year-old man has been worried about having contracted human immunodeficiency virus (HIV). He has undergone repeated tests for HIV, but is not reassured by the negative results.
3. A 35-year-old man was admitted via the A&E department with complaints suggestive of acute abdomen. He had a number of scars on his abdomen. A staff nurse remembered seeing him in another hospital with similar complaints. When confronted he became aggressive and discharged himself against medical advice.
4. A 45-year-old man was found wandering the streets aimlessly in Edinburgh and was taken to the A&E department by the police. He could not remember his name or any other details. Later he was identified as a missing person from London. He was about to be arrested in London for fraud.
5. A 16-year-old student is referred by her GP. Her family members are concerned that she spends hours in front of the mirror examining her nose. She is convinced that her nose is deformed and is refusing to go to school. She has been saving money to get plastic surgery done on her nose. There is no obvious deformity.

6.23 Stress-related disorders

Options

a. Agoraphobia
b. Briquet's syndrome
c. Conversion disorder
d. Factitious illness
e. Generalised anxiety disorder
f. Hypochondriasis
g. Panic disorder
h. Social phobia
i. PTSD
j. Simple phobia

Lead in

Match each presentation below with one diagnosis:

Presentations

1. A 24-year-old male presents with easy fatigability, poor sleep, difficulty concentrating, with anxiety and apprehension of something untoward going to happen.
2. An 18-year-old student presents with anxiety attacks, diaphoresis and palpitations when eating in restaurants, using public transport and attending parties.
3. A 26-year-old female was admitted to the medical ward for evaluation of sudden onset of aphonia. Her partner died in an accident 2 days previously. Physical examination and investigations were normal.
4. A 33-year-old woman had numerous admissions to the orthopaedic ward for evaluation of severe lower back pain with no relief from analgesics. All investigations were normal. During a psychiatric assessment she insists that only surgery could cure her and pleadingly asks if this could be recommended to the orthopaedic team.
5. A 23-year-old female was admitted with a history of depression and attempted suicide. She gives a history of dysphoria, headaches, neck pain, dysmenorrhoea and menorrhagia. She also complains of 'pins and needles' in her extremities, poor appetite, nausea and loose stools. She seems to be in distress during the examination, complaining that her lower back hurts. Her physical examination and investigations were all normal.

6.26 Women's disorders

Options

a. A disproportionately larger number consult their GP
b. Belief that the child is evil
c. Breast tenderness, abdominal discomfort and feeling of distension
d. Flushing, sweating and vaginal dryness
e. Occurs in 30–80% of women
f. Occurs in 10% of women postpartum
g. Onset within 1–2 weeks postpartum
h. Peaks 3–4 days postpartum
i. Tiredness, irritability and anxiety more often than mood change
j. Triad of irritability, labile mood and confusion

Lead in

Choose two features each for the following disorders:

Disorders

1. Postpartum psychosis
2. Postnatal depression
3. Premenstrual syndrome
4. Menopause
5. Maternity blues

Answers

6.1 Alcohol and drugs

1-g. Extradural haemorrhage (OM4-440).
2-f. Delirium tremens (OTP4-546).
3-d. Alcoholic hallucinosis (OTP4-547).
4-c. Alcoholic memory blackout (CTP7-957).
5-b. Alcohol–disulfiram interaction (OTP4-555).

6.2 Anorexia

1-a. Bradycardia with hypotension (CPS7-492).
2-e. Metabolic acidosis. Vomiting causes metabolic alkalosis.
3-d. Low T3 and high growth hormone. Also low oestrogen, low progesterone and high cortisol.
4-i. Raised. Also hypercarotenaemia and high beta-hydroxybutyrate.
5-h. Normocytic normochromic anaemia and thrombocytopenia, with Hb = 9–12 g/l. Pancytopaenia is common in severe cases (Stein & Wilkinson-870; CPS7-492).

6.3 Anxiety disorders

1-f. Panic disorder, moderate (ICD-10).
2-d. Generalised anxiety disorder.
3-a. Acute stress reaction.
4-i. Social phobia.
5-c. Agoraphobia.

6.4 Bereavement

1-g. Severe depressive episode (OTP4-208; CTP7-1976).
2-i. Stage two of bereavement (CTP7-1975).
3-d. Delayed grief (OTP4-209).
4-b. Anniversary reaction (CTP7-1975).
5-f. Prolonged grief.

6.5 Clinical diagnoses

1-j. Somatisation disorder (ICD-10).
2-g. Hypochondriasis.
3-i. Schizophrenia.
4-c. Depressive episode.
5-d. Emotionally unstable personality disorder – borderline type.

6.6 Clinical features

1-a. Anorexia nervosa.
2-i. Pica.
3-f. Mania with psychotic symptoms.
4-c. Body dysmorphic disorder.
5-e. Diogenes syndrome.

6.7 Clinical features of anxiety disorders

1-c. Agoraphobia with panic disorder (ICD-10; DSM-IV; CPS7-450).
2-j. Social phobia.
3-i. PTSD.
4-b. Adjustment disorder – brief depressive reaction.
5-h. Panic disorder.

6.8 Clinical pictures

1-i. Secondary gain.
2-j. Somatosensory amplification.
3-f. Hysterical blindness.
4-h. Non-cardiac chest pain.
5-e. Dyspareunia.

6.9 Clinical syndromes

1-e. HIV encephalopathy.
2-f. PTSD.
3-g. Rapid-cycling bipolar disorder.
4-a. Adjustment disorder with anxiety.
5-i. Bipolar II disorder.

6.10 Complications of anorexia

1-b. Hypophosphataemia – associated with cardiac arrest during refeeding.
2-j. Osteoporosis – can cause wedge fractures of thoracic spine and disturbed breathing mechanics.
3-c. Hypofolataemia – can cause degeneration of the dorsal columns of the spinal cord.
4-e. Hypokalaemia – can complicate excessive vomiting.
5-f. Hyponatraemia – if rapidly corrected, can lead to central pontine myelinolysis.

6.11 Culture-bound syndromes

1-f. Latah (CTP7-463; NOTP-1061; DSM-IV).
2-e. Koro.
3-g. Pibloktoq.
4-j. Windigo.
5-c. Brain Fag.

6.12 Diagnosis of anxiety disorders

1-d. Generalised anxiety disorder.
2-b. Agoraphobia.
3-h. Social phobia.
4-g. PTSD.
5-i. Conversion disorder (OTP4-254).

6.13 Diagnosis of eating disorders

1-b. Anorexia nervosa (ICD-10).
2-g. Hyperthyroidism. May mimic eating disorders. Also, exophthalmia, high T3 high T4 and low TSH. (OM4-542).
3-a. Addison's disease. Low cortisol, ACTH > 300 ng/l at 9.00 and 22.00 hrs. Causes include autoimmune, insulin-dependent diabetes mellitus (IDDM), pernicious anaemia (OM4-552).
4-c. Bulimia nervosa (ICD-10).
5-d. Coeliac disease. Prolamin intolerance causes villous atrophy and malabsorption, resulting in steatorrhoea, vitamin deficiencies, weight loss and bloating. Prolamin is an alcohol-soluble protein found in wheat, barley etc. (OM4-522).

6.14 Dissociative disorders

1-c. Fugue. Sudden unexpected travel away from home or one's place of work with inability to recall one's past (OTP4-264).
2-e. Multiple personality disorder. Presence of two or more distinct identities or personality states that take control of the person's behaviour and an inability to recall important information (ICD-10).
3-g. Munchausen syndrome.
4-i. Retrograde amnesia.
5-f. Munchausen syndrome by proxy.

6.15 Drug intoxication and withdrawal

1-f,g,d. Pupillary dilatation, seizures, nausea (CTP7-1045).
2-a,c,i. Dysphoric mood, increased appetite, vivid dreams (CTP7-1004).
3-b,e,h. Inco-ordination, nystagmus, slurred speech (CTP7-1029).
4-f,j,d. Pupillary dilation, yawning, nausea (CTP7-1045).
5-b,e,h. Inco-ordination, nystagmus, slurred speech (CTP7-076).

6.16 Epidemiology of suicide

1-e. 3:1 (OTP4-509).
2-i. Social classes I and V (OTP4-509).
3-g. Depressive disorders in 36–90% and personality disorders in 5–44% of those who commit suicide (OTP4-511).
4-b. 100 times (OTP4-507).
5-d. 66%. Two-thirds see their GP in the previous month and 40% in the previous week. One-quarter sees a psychiatrist, of whom half see a psychiatrist in the week before suicide (OTP4-507).

6.17 Late-onset schizophrenia

1-a. Approximately 25% (Lawlor).
2-d. Later.
3-j. Women.
4-g. Lower.
5-e. Less impaired.

6.18 Paraphilias

1-i. Transsexualism (ICD-10).
2-a. Dual-role transvestism.
3-d. Fetishistic transvestism.
4-b. Exhibitionism.
5-j. Voyeurism.

6.19 Personality disorders

1-i,j. Paranoid, schizoid (also schizotypal. It is not in ICD-10).
2-a,c,e,g. Antisocial, borderline personality disorder, histrionic, narcissistic.
3-b,h. Avoidant, obsessive–compulsive (also dependent).
4-c,h,a,g,b Borderline personality disorder, obsessive–compulsive, antisocial, narcissistic, avoidant. ICD-10 uses alternative terms, e.g. emotionally unstable–borderline type, dissocial, anankastic and anxious–avoidant. Narcissistic is not included in ICD-10.
5-f. Mixed personality disorder. Instead DSM-IV uses personality disorder not otherwise specified.

6.20 Personality traits

1-a. Allusive thinking.
2-c. Failure to plan ahead.
3-h. Parsimony.
4-g. Impressionistic speech.
5-d. Feelings of emptiness and boredom.

6.21 Sexual dysfunction

1-d,h,b. Performance anxiety; squeeze technique or fluoxetine (OTP4-596).
2-i,g. Traumatic early sexual experience; sensate focus techniques and graduated vaginal dilation (OTP4-597).
3-a,c. Diabetes mellitus; papaverine (OTP4-594).
4-j,e. Trazodone; phenylephrine (BNF47; CTP7-1605).
5-b,f. Fluoxetine; sensate focus techniques and graduated masturbation (OTP4-596).

6.22 Somatoform disorders

1-i. Somatization disorder (OTP4-257).
2-e. Hypochondriacal disorder (ICD-10).
3-g. Munchausen syndrome (OTP4-475).
4-c. Dissociative fugue state (ICD-10).
5-a. Body dysmorphic disorder (OTP4-258).

6.23 Stress-related disorders

1-e. Generalised anxiety disorder. Differentiate from PTSD by absence of history of severe inciting trauma and panic disorder by no discrete attacks of panic (ICD-10).
2-h. Social phobia.
3-c. Conversion disorder.
4-d. Factitious disorder.
5-b. Briquet's syndrome (somatisation disorder).

6.24 Substance misuse

1-c. Delirium tremens. The classical triad is confusion, tremor and vivid hallucinations (Edwards-95).
2-i. Opiate overdose. Enlarged lymph nodes may be secondary to abscesses from injecting.
3-e. Intra-cranial haematoma. Hemisomatognosia (Lishman-68).
4-j. Wernicke's encephalopathy. The full triad does not always occur. One should have a high index of suspicion in a heavy drinker and treat promptly (Edwards-103).
5-g. Korsakoff's psychosis. This may occur insidiously with or without a clear history of Wernicke's encephalopathy (Edwards-105).

6.25 Uncommon syndromes

1-d. Couvade syndrome (Enoch & Ball).
2-h. Ganser's syndrome.
3-b. Capgras' syndrome.
4-i. Othello syndrome.
5-e. de Clerambult's syndrome.

6.26 Women's disorders

1-b, g. Belief that the child is evil. Onset within 1–2 weeks postpartum (OTP4-499).

2-f, i. Tiredness, irritability and anxiety more often than mood change. Occurs in 10% of women postpartum.

3-c, e. Breast tenderness, abdominal discomfort and feeling of distension. Occurs in 30–80% of women.

4-d, a. Flushing, sweating and vaginal dryness. A disproportionately larger number consult their GP during their middle ages, including the perimenopausal years.

5-j, h. Triad of irritability, labile mood and confusion. Peaks 3–4 days postpartum.

7. Organic psychiatry

7.1   Abnormalities of movement

Options

a. Akathisia
b. Catalepsy
c. Cataplexy
d. Huntington's disease
e. Dystonia
f. Myoclonus fit
g. Narcolepsy
h. Stereotypy
i. Tardive dystonia
j. Tardive dyskinesia

Lead in

Select one option each to describe the following scenarios:

Scenarios

1. A 60-year-old female has facial grimaces and movements of her mouth with occasional protruding movements of her tongue. She has been on antipsychotics for the past 30 years.
2. A 20-year-old male has occasional episodes of collapse accompanied by loss of muscle tone. This often occurs when he is laughing.
3. A 24-year-old male develops involuntary painful protrusion of his tongue an hour after he is given haloperidol.
4. A young manager gets recurrent irresistible brief episodes of sleep during the day, even while attending important meetings, despite sleeping well in the night.
5. A middle-aged male presents with sudden jerky movements of the arms. He also has a dysarthria, has recently developed changes in his gait and complains of feeling depressed. His father died at the age of 50 and had similar symptoms.

7.2   Abnormal movements

Options

a. Acute dystonia
b. Akathisia
c. Athetosis
d. Automatism
e. Cataplexy
f. Catatonia
g. Chorea
h. Hemiballismus
i. Myoclonus
j. Sydenham's chorea

Lead in

Match the presentations with one option each:

Presentations

1. A 72-year-old male recovering from left-sided hemiplegia following an intracranial haemorrhage develops sudden aimless and vigorous movements of the trunk and left arm.

2. A middle-aged woman complains of an inner restlessness in her legs and a compulsion to move her legs. She was recently started on haloperidol 5 mg daily for paranoid psychosis.

3. A 20-year-old student is brought with a four-day history of not speaking, eating or even moving. Over the past few months he has become withdrawn and has had deteriorating grades. He stopped attending college a month ago. He does not appear to be hallucinating.

4. A 45-year-old male was admitted with a one-year history of dizziness, anxiety, apathy and memory impairment. He has brief asynchronous muscular jerks of the extremities.

5. A 32-year-old secretary presents with a history of sudden falls, when she drops anything that she is holding at the time. These episodes occur when she is emotionally excited. Her supervisor is cross with her because he has seen her sleeping on her desk on many occasions.

7.3   Alzheimer's disease

Options

a. Aluminium
b. Depression
c. Early onset
d. Female gender
e. Head injury
f. Hypomania
g. Late onset
h. Male gender
i. Oestrogen
j. Smoking

Lead in

Choose one option each that best fits the statements below:

Statements

1. Alzheimer's disease is less common in this gender.
2. This type of Alzheimer's disease is associated with a stronger familial risk.
3. This is often a prodromal feature of Alzheimer's disease.
4. This has been associated with both an increased and decreased risk of Alzheimer's disease.
5. While some earlier studies showed a possible link between this and Alzheimer's disease it is now accepted that it is neither necessary nor sufficient to cause Alzheimer's disease.

7.4   Cerebral arteries

Options

a. Anterior cerebral artery (bilateral)
b. Anterior cerebral artery (unilateral)
c. Carotid artery
d. Circle of Willis
e. Circular artery
f. Communicating artery
g. Internal auditory artery
h. Middle cerebral artery
i. Posterior inferior cerebellar artery (PICA)
j. Subclavian artery proximal to the ipsilateral vertebral artery

Lead in

Identify one cerebral artery each, the occlusion of which would cause the following symptoms:

Symptoms

1. Contralateral hemiplegia and sensory loss, mainly in the face and arm
2. Contralateral weakness of the leg and milder symptoms in the arm, with face spared
3. Vomiting, nystagmus on looking to the side of the lesion, ipsilateral Horner's syndrome
4. Brainstem ischaemia following arm exertion, causing difference in BP of > 20 mmHg between the arms
5. Akinetic mute state

7.5   Cranial nerve lesions

Options

a. Bilateral glossopharyngeal nerve lesion
b. Bilateral vagus nerve lesion
c. Bilateral temporal hemianopia
d. Downwards and outwards
e. Homonymous hemianopia
f. Left lower motor neuron lesion of the accessory nerve
g. Right upper motor neuron lesion of the accessory nerve
h. Upwards and inwards
i. Unilateral lower motor neuron lesion of facial nerve
j. Unilateral upper motor neuron lesion of facial nerve

Lead in

Find one option each for the following lesions and symptoms:

Lesions and symptoms

1. Optic chiasma lesion produces ___.
2. In oculomotor nerve palsy, the eye is deviated ___.
3. Bell's palsy is caused by ___.
4. Inability to elevate the palate voluntarily suggests ___.
5. Weakness of the right sternocleidomastoid and left trapezius muscles suggests ___.

7.6 Creutzfeldt–Jakob disease

Options

a. Equally prevalent in variant and sporadic CJD
b. Longer in variant CJD than sporadic CJD
c. More frequent in sporadic CJD than variant CJD
d. More frequent in variant CJD than sporadic CJD
e. Older in sporadic CJD than variant CJD
f. Same age in sporadic and variant CJD
g. Same duration in sporadic and variant CJD
h. Same in sporadic and variant CJD
i. Shorter in variant CJD than sporadic CJD
j. Younger in sporadic CJD than variant CJD

Lead in

Select one option each for the followings aspects of CJD:

Aspects

1. Typical age of onset
2. Typical duration of illness (from onset until death)
3. Prevalence of psychiatric features at disease onset
4. Prevalence of periodic complexes on electroencephalogram
5. Prevalence of disease-specific abnormalities on MRI

7.7 Delirium

Options

a. Alcohol intoxication
b. Diabetic ketoacidosis
c. Extradural haemorrhage
d. Hepatic encephalopathy
e. Hypoglycaemia
f. Meningitis
g. Sjögren's syndrome
h. Subarachnoid haemorrhage
i. Tetanus
j. Wernicke's encephalopathy

Lead in

Choose one diagnosis each for the following presentations:

Presentations

1. A 56-year-old man with a history of chronic heavy alcohol consumption presents with a one-week history of drowsiness, confusion, lethargy and slurred speech. His breath smells sweet.

2. A 37-year-old female is brought to the A&E department with a sudden onset of severe headache, vomiting, collapse and fluctuating consciousness. On examination, she has a stiff neck and papilloedema.

3. A 25-year-old woman presents with a 24-hour history of headache, photophobia, stiff neck, vomiting and fever. She has tachycardia, hypotension, papilloedema and skin rash. Her cerebrospinal fluid (CSF) is turbid with polymorphs and low glucose.

4. A 60-year-old man with a history of insulin-dependent diabetes mellitus is brought to the A&E department with complaints of increasing tremulousness, drowsiness, confusion and sweating since that morning. He had a seizure at noon.

5. A 35-year-old man with a history of chronic alcohol abuse is brought to the A&E department with confusion, vomiting and headache. On examination he has ataxia, lateral rectus palsy and sluggish pupils.

7.8 Dementias

Options

a. Alzheimer's disease
b. Alcoholic dementia
c. Chronic subdural haematoma
d. Dementia in Creutzfeldt–Jakob disease
e. Dementia in Huntington's disease
f. Dementia in Pick's disease
g. Dementia with Lewy bodies
h. Depressive pseudodementia
i. Multi-infarct dementia
j. Normal pressure hydrocephalus

Lead in

Choose one diagnosis each for the following scenarios:

Scenarios

1. A 60-year-old man is referred with a history of worsening memory and urinary incontinence. He has a broad-based, short-stepped gait. A CT scan showed ventricular enlargement out of proportion with cortical atrophy and periventricular signal change.
2. A GP refers an 85-year-old man with a history of seeing 'strange' things, dizziness, repeated falls, and occasional loss of consciousness. The GP prescribed risperidone, which caused several severe extrapyramidal side effects.
3. Brought by his wife, a 68-year-old man complained of depression and confusion in the night for the past 4 months. He is fine some days, but very anxious other days. On examination, he has brisk reflexes, spastic weakness of left lower limb and an extensor plantar response.
4. A GP is concerned that a 60-year-old woman who lives alone has become very restless and quite disinhibited lately. A CT scan shows 'knife blade atrophy' of temporal and frontal lobes.
5. A daughter brings her 58-year-old mother, who lives with her, with a history of becoming increasingly withdrawn and flattened in mood over the past few months. Lately, her memory has been deteriorating. She was uncooperative for a MMSE.

7.9　Diagnosis of sleep disorders

Options

a. Catalepsy
b. Cataplexy
c. Kleine–Levin syndrome
d. Kluver–Bucy syndrome
e. Narcolepsy
f. Nightmares
g. Night terrors
h. Pickwickian syndrome
i. Prader–Willi syndrome
j. Somnambulism

Lead in

Select one option each that corresponds best to the descriptions below:

Descriptions

1. Periodic somnolence with intense hunger.
2. Occurs in 15% of children and 2–5% of adults, predominantly in males, and is associated with enuresis and low levels of arousal.
3. An elderly obese man who snores a lot complains of daytime somnolence. His wife is concerned that he stops breathing regularly during sleep.
4. Occurs in stages 3 and 4 of sleep, is associated with autonomic arousal, and followed by amnesia for the episode. There is often a strong family history.
5. A 20-year-old male who has irresistible attacks of daytime somnolence, leading to several short episodes of sleep associated with hypnagogic hallucinations.

7.10 Disorders of speech

Options

a. Cerebellar lesions
b. Disorder of Wernicke's area
c. Extrapyramidal lesions
d. Hysterical
e. Laryngeal lesions
f. Lesions of Broca's area
g. Lower motor neuron lesions
h. Myasthenia gravis
i. Upper motor neuron lesions
j. Vocal cord paralysis

Lead in

Match one option each with the following dysarthrias:

Dysarthrias

1. Slow, slurred, monotonous, low-pitched speech without inflections. The words are often trailed at the end of sentences
2. Slurred and indistinct speech with a nasal quality
3. Slow, slurred, monotonous, high-pitched speech
4. Slow, slurred and scanning speech
5. Worsening of dysarthria as the day progresses

7.11 Endocrine disorders

Options

a. Acute porphyria
b. Addison's disease
c. Cushing's syndrome
d. Diabetes insipidus
e. Diabetes mellitus
f. Hyperparathyroidism
g. Hyperthyroidism
h. Hypothyroidism
i. Phaeochromocytoma
j. Psychogenic polydipsia

Lead in

Identify one disorder each that best fits with the following presentations:

Presentations

1. Anxiety, palpitations, loss of weight and tachycardia
2. Weakness, loss of appetite and weight, apathy, hyponatraemia and hyperkalaemia
3. Polydipsia, polyuria, low urine osmolality and low plasma osmolality
4. Paroxysmal palpitations, sweating and anxiety with hypertension
5. Lack of initiative, depression, increased thirst and insidious change of personality

7.12 Epilepsy

Options

a. Arching of the back with asymmetrical jerks of limbs
b. Can have secondary generalisation
c. Consciousness may be fully retained
d. Decreased post-ictal serum prolactin
e. Electroencephalogram (EEG) shows generalized 2–4 Hz spike and slow wave activity
f. EEG shows multispikes followed by multispikes and slow waves
g. Loss of awareness is a cardinal feature
h. May start from a focal lesion
i. Seizures differ from attack to attack
j. Stereotypical seizure pattern

Lead in

Find the features of the types of epilepsies:

Types of epilepsies

1. Absence seizures (3)
2. Complex partial seizures (4)
3. Grand mal seizures (3)
4. Pseudoseizures (3)
5. Simple partial seizures (4)

7.13 Features of dementias

Options

a. Atrophy of striatum
b. Early abnormal movements of hands, shoulders and face
c. Early cerebellar ataxia
d. Focal signs of parietal lobe dysfunction
e. Intracytoplasmic neuronal inclusions
f. Neurofibrillary tangles
g. Numerous infarcts in basal ganglia or cortex
h. PrP plaques
i. Signs of parkinsonism
j. Stepwise deterioration

Lead in

Select one neuropathological feature and one clinical feature each for the following conditions:

Conditions

1. Huntington's disease
2. Alzheimer's disease
3. Dementia with Lewy bodies
4. Sporadic Creutzfeldt–Jakob disease
5. Multi-infarct dementia

7.14 Human immunodeficiency virus

Options

a. Adjustment disorder
b. Anxiety disorder
c. Cortical dementia
d. Depression
e. Delirium
f. HIV-associated dementia
g. Mania
h. Psychosis
i. Subclinical cognitive impairment
j. Subcortical dementia

Lead in

Select one option each for the following conditions (use one option only once):

Conditions

1. The regional type of dementia seen in patients with HIV
2. Most common psychiatric diagnosis in patients with HIV
3. Up to one-third of patients with HIV may suffer from this affective disorder
4. A common manifestation of involvement of the right frontal lobe
5. The most common dementia in patients with AIDS

7.15 Memory disorders

Options

a. Adjustment disorder
b. Alzheimer's disease
c. Amnesic syndrome
d. CADASIL (Cerebral Autosomal Dominant Arteriopathy with Subcortical Infarcts and Leukoencephalopathy)
e. Dissociative amnesia
f. Fugue
g. Korsakoff's syndrome
h. Lewy body dementia
i. Multi-infarct dementia
j. Pseudodementia

Lead in

Match each of the following presentations with one of the options:

Presentations

1. A 77-year-old man presents with fluctuating, progressive memory decline. He also has a history of hypertension and falls.
2. The police bring a middle-aged male to A&E. He appears unable to remember his personal details. He is otherwise well and all investigations are normal.
3. A 67-year-old woman presents with memory deficits following the death of her husband 2 months previously. She also complains of lethargy, disturbed sleep and weight loss.
4. A 64-year-old woman presents with cognitive impairment, particularly confusion and bizarre behaviour towards the late evening. On examination, she has hypersalivation and hypertonia. These are exacerbated following antipsychotic therapy.
5. A 55-year-old male presents to the clinic with a complaint of cognitive impairment. He gives a history of migraines with aura and episodes of muscular weakness.

7.16 Metabolic disturbances

Options

a. Hypercalcaemia
b. Hyperglycaemia
c. Hyperkalaemia
d. Hypermagnesaemia
e. Hypernatraemia
f. Hypocalcaemia
g. Hypoglycaemia
h. Hypokalaemia
i. Hyponatraemia
j. Uremia

Lead in

Identify one metabolic disturbance for each of the following scenarios:

Scenarios

1. A 30-year-old woman complains of weakness in her arms and legs after a fall. There is a long history of anorexia, lethargy, constipation and abdominal distension.
2. A 36-year-old diabetic man presents to casualty with nausea and muscle cramps. He appears to be lethargic. He recently became depressed and last week he commenced fluoxetine 20 mg daily.
3. A 32-year-old man with chronic schizophrenia commenced clozapine 4 weeks ago. Now he becomes agitated, confused, and complains of abdominal pain.
4. A 53-year-old woman with alcohol dependence visits the emergency GP complaining of severe anxiety. History reveals she drank a bottle of whisky 16 hours ago.
5. A 25-year-old man with sarcoidosis complains of increased thirst, low mood and he thinks his wife is trying to poison him.

7.17 Neurodegenerative disorders

Options

a. Alzheimer's dementia
b. Corticobasal degeneration
c. Frontotemporal dementia
d. Huntington's disease
e. Hydrocephalic dementia
f. Lewy body dementia
g. Pick's disease
h. Progressive supranuclear palsy
i. Vascular dementia
j. Wilson's disease

Lead in

Select one option each for the following descriptions:

Descriptions

1. Dementia associated with fluctuating cognition and sensitivity to antipsychotic medication
2. Genetically transmitted neurodegenerative disorder primarily affecting the striatum
3. Neurodegenerative disorder affecting the brainstem and basal ganglia
4. Dementia characterised by personality alteration, poor insight, poor judgement and preservation of visuospatial skills
5. Dementia associated with gait disturbance and incontinence

7.5 Cranial nerve lesions

I-c. Bilateral temporal hemianopia. Lesions beyond the optic chiasma produce homonymous hemianopia (OM4-458).

2-d. Downwards and outwards. The eye is abducted by the lateral rectus muscle and depressed by the superior oblique muscle (NFP-31).

3-i. Unilateral lower motor neuron lesion of facial nerve (NFP-37).

4-b. Bilateral vagus nerve lesion (NFP-45).

5-g. Right upper motor neuron lesion of accessory nerve. Peripheral accessory nerve lesions cause ipsilateral sternocleidomastoid and ipsilateral trapezius weakness (NFP-46).

7.6 Creutzfeldt–Jakob disease

I-e. Older in sporadic CJD than variant CJD (Spencer *et al*, 2002; CJD).

2-b. Longer in variant CJD than sporadic CJD.

3-d. More frequent in variant CJD than sporadic CJD.

4-c. More frequent in sporadic CJD than variant CJD.

5-d. More frequent in variant CJD than sporadic CJD.

7.7 Delirium

I-d. Hepatic encephalopathy (OM4-504).

2-h. Subarachnoid haemorrhage. Caused by rupture of Berry's aneurysm in 70% (OM4-438).

3-f. Meningitis. The CSF is normal in tetanus (OM4-442).

4-e. Hypoglycaemia. The commonest endocrine emergency (OM4-536).

5-j. Wernicke's encephalopathy (OM4-712).

7.8 Dementias

I-j. Normal pressure hydrocephalus (OTP4-428).

2-g. Dementia with Lewy bodies. They are extremely sensitive to EPSE (OTP4-625).

3-i. Multi-infarct dementia (OTP4-626; ICD-10).

4-f. Dementia in Pick's disease (OTP4-420; ICD-10).

5-h. Depressive pseudodementia. Depressive symptoms precede cognitive decline. Non-cooperation is common (OTP4-418).

7.9 Diagnosis of sleep disorders

I-c. Kleine–Levin syndrome (Lishman-688).

2-j. Somnambulism.

3-h. Pickwickian syndrome.

4-g. Night terrors.

5-e. Narcolepsy.

7.10 Disorders of speech

1-c. Extrapyramidal lesions (NFP-16–17).
2-g. Lower motor neuron lesions – resulting in bulbar palsy (OM4-466).
3-i. Upper motor neuron lesions – resulting in pseudobulbar palsy. The tongue is small, contracted and lies in the floor of the mouth. Also called "Donald Duck" dysarthria.
4-a. Cerebellar lesions. Speech is broken down into syllables and spoken with varying force.
5-h. Myasthenia gravis.

7.11 Endocrine disorders

1-g. Hyperthyroidism (Lishman-507).
2-b. Addison's disease.
3-j. Psychogenic polydipsia.
4-i. Phaeochromocytoma.
5-f. Hyperparathyroidism.

7.12 Epilepsy

1-e,g,j. EEG shows generalised 2–4 Hz spike and slow wave activity; loss of awareness is a cardinal feature; stereotypical seizure pattern (Lishman-237; CTP7-261).
2-b,g,h,j. Can have secondary generalisation; loss of awareness is a cardinal feature; may start from a focal lesion; stereotypical seizure pattern.
3-f,g,j. EEG shows multispikes followed by multispikes and slow waves; loss of awareness is a cardinal feature; stereotypical seizure pattern.
4-a,c,i. Arching of the back with asymmetrical jerks of limbs; consciousness may be fully retained; seizures differ from attack to attack.
5-b,h,c,j. Can have secondary generalisation; may start from a focal lesion; consciousness may be fully retained; stereotypical seizure pattern.

7.13 Features of dementias

1-a,b. Atrophy of striatum; early abnormal movements of hands, shoulders and face.
2-f,d. Neurofibrillary tangles; focal signs of parietal lobe dysfunction.
3-e,i. Intracytoplasmic neuronal inclusions; signs of parkinsonism.
4-h,c. PrP plaques; early cerebellar ataxia.
5-g,j. Numerous infarcts in basal ganglia or cortex; stepwise deterioration.

7.14 HIV

1-j. Subcortical dementia. HIV-associated dementia is a subcortical dementia affecting subcortical and frontostriatal areas (Di Rocco & Werner 1999).

2-e. Delirium. May be undetected in up to 30 percent of cases.

3-d. Depression (OTP4-493).

4-g. Mania. Mania in patients with HIV may be related to premorbid bipolar disorder, brain lesions from HIV, opportunistic infections, neoplasms or medication.

5-f. HIV-associated dementia.

7.15 Memory disorders

1-i. Multi-infarct dementia.

2-f. Fugue.

3-j. Pseudodementia.

4-h. Lewy body dementia.

5-d. CADASIL. Occurs in young adults. Presents with migraines, mood disturbances, focal neurological deficits, strokes, and dementia.

7.16 Metabolic disturbances

1-h. Hypokalaemia. Causes include renal tubular acidosis and Cushing's disease. Such complaints may be mistaken for hysteria (Lishman-507; MPG7).

2-i. Hyponatraemia. The mention of diabetes is a red herring. The key factor here is fluoxetine. All antidepressants can cause hyponatraemia, especially SSRIs.

3-b. Hyperglycaemia. Clozapine can cause hyperglycaemia through insulin resistance. Ketoacidosis may cause abdominal pain and confusion.

4-g. Hypoglycaemia. Alcohol-induced hypoglycaemia typically occurs in alcohol dependence, 6–36 hours after a large intake.

5-a. Hypercalcaemia. Sarcoidosis is associated with hypercalcaemia, which can manifest with depression and paranoia.

7.17 Neurodegenerative disorders

1-f. Lewy body dementia (Yudofsky & Hales-953).

2-d. Huntington's disease.

3-h. Progressive supranuclear palsy. Characterised by supranuclear gaze palsy, pseudobulbar palsy, rigidity and dementia.

4-c. Frontotemporal dementia.

5-e. Hydrocephalic dementia or normal pressure hydrocephalus.

7.18 Neuroendocrine disorders

1-e. Diabetes mellitus (Lishman-507).
2-a. Acute porphyria.
3-c. Cushing's syndrome.
4-h. Hypothyroidism.
5-d. Diabetes insipidus.

7.19 Organic psychiatry

1-j. Visual hallucinations.
2-b. Confabulation.
3-g. Pica.
4-c. Incontinence.
5-a. Abulia.

7.20 Organic syndromes

1-c. Empty high spirits and a boisterous manner (Lishman-76, 512, 745).
2-f. Hyperactivity and learning disability.
3-b. Constipation, poor appetite and impaired taste.
4-e. Forgetfulness, slowing of mental activity and gait disturbances.
5-h. Hypogonadism, mild impairment of intelligence, and impaired verbal abilities in comparison to the non-verbal ones.

7.21 Presentation of dementias

1-c. Dementia in Creutzfeldt–Jakob disease.
2-g. Dementia in Pick's disease.
3-b. Dementia in Alzheimer's disease.
4-a. Delirium.
5-j. Vascular dementia.

7.22 Sleep disorders

1-c,e. Cataplexy; hypnopompic hallucinations (DSM-IV-551).
2-g,j. More common in females; occurs during REM sleep.
3-a,i. Amnesia for the episode; occurs in the first 3rd of sleep.
4-a,i. Amnesia for the episode; occurs in the first 3rd of sleep.
5-f,h. More common in males; more common and worse in the elderly.

7.23 Speech disorders

1-b. Echolalia (Sims-159).
2-g. Paragrammatism (Sims-159).
3-h. Perseveration (Sims-55).
4-a. Aphonia (Sims-158).
5-c. Flight of ideas (Sims-137).

7.24 Viral infections

1-i.   *Toxoplasma gondii*. May present with focal or diffuse cognitive and affective disturbance (Yudofsky & Hales-787).

2-c.   *Cryptococcus neoformans*.

3-d.   Cytomegalovirus. Presents with encephalitis, retinitis and peripheral neuropathy and demyelination.

4-e.   Herpes simplex virus. This may manifest as temporal lobe encephalitis or encephalomyelitis in immune-deficient patients.

5-j.   Tuberculous meningitis. Biopsy aids diagnosis.

8. Investigations

8.1 Choice of investigations

Options

a. Adoption studies
b. Case reports
c. Cross-sectional studies
d. Interventional studies
e. Postmortem studies
f. Retrospective studies
g. Studies of army conscripts
h. Studies of cohorts of unmedicated patients
i. Studies from home movies
j. Family studies

Lead in

Choose one setting each for studying the following aspects of schizophrenia:

Aspects

1. Identification of premorbid neuromotor abnormalities
2. Identification of premorbid intellectual deficits
3. Dissociation of genetic and environmental factors
4. Characterisation of the natural history of the disorder
5. Efficacy of treatment

8.2   Cognitive assessment

Options

a. Attention
b. Consciousness
c. Episodic memory
d. Executive frontal dysfunction
e. Intelligence quotient
f. Occipital lobe function
g. Parietal lobe function
h. Premorbid intelligence
i. Semantic memory
j. Working memory

Lead in

Choose one area of cognition that best corresponds to each cognitive test below:

Cognitive tests

1. Letter- and category-based fluency
2. Serial subtraction
3. Object naming and defining the meaning of words
4. Memory for events specific to time and place, and unique to each individual
5. Solving arithmetical problems in the head

8.3 Cognitive function tests

Options

a. Brain damage
b. Executive function
c. Language
d. Memory
e. Non-verbal intelligence
f. Parietal lobe function
g. Perception
h. Pre-morbid intelligence
i. Sensory inattention
j. Vigilance

Lead in

Choose one function each assessed by the following tests:

Tests

1. Raven's Progressive Matrices
2. Rey–Osterrieth Test
3. Wisconsin Card Sorting Test
4. National Adult Reading Test
5. Halstead–Reitan Battery

8.4   EEG changes

Options

a. Creutzfeldt–Jakob disease
b. Depressive pseudodementia
c. Focal structural lesion
d. Generalised anxiety state
e. Herpes simplex encephalitis
f. Huntington's chorea
g. Metabolic encephalopathy
h. Myoclonic epilepsy
i. Subacute sclerosing panencephalitis
j. Typical absence seizure

Lead in

Select one option each for the following EEG changes:

EEG changes

1. Generalised theta or delta wave activities
2. 3 Hz bilateral, symmetrical spike-and-wave activity
3. Focal slow-wave activity
4. Generalised multiple spike-and-wave activity
5. Periodic, generalized 1–2 Hz sharp waves over low amplitude and slow background

8.5   EEG waves

Options

a. Alpha waves
b. Beta waves
c. Delta waves
d. Focal activity
e. Gamma waves
f. Irregular waves
g. Omega waves
h. Slow waves
i. Spike waves
j. Theta waves

Lead in

Identify the following EEG waves:

Frequencies

1. 4–8 Hz, which occurs during sleep
2. 8–13 Hz
3. <4 Hz
4. >13 Hz
5. That increases when relaxed with eyes closed

8.6   Endocrine investigations

Options

a. 24-hour urinary VMA
b. Dexamethasone suppression test
c. Fasting plasma glucose
d. Oral glucose tolerance test with GH measurement
e. Plasma and urine osmolality
f. Plasma aldosterone and renin measurement
g. Parathyroid hormone
h. Short adrenocorticotropic hormone (ACTH) stimulation test (Short Synacthen test)
i. Thyroid antibodies
j. Thyroid-stimulating hormone

Lead in

Select one investigation each for the diagnosis of the following conditions:

Conditions

1. Cushing's disease
2. Phaeochromocytoma
3. Hypothyroidism
4. Diabetes mellitus
5. Grave's disease

8.7   Endocrine tests

Options

a. 24-hour urinary VMA
b. Dexamethasone suppression test
c. Fasting plasma glucose
d. Oral glucose tolerance test with growth hormone levels
e. Plasma and urine osmolality
f. Plasma aldosterone and renin measurement
g. Parathyroid hormone
h. Short ACTH stimulation test (Short Synacthen test)
i. Thyroid antibodies
j. Thyroid stimulating hormone

Lead in

Select one investigation each for the diagnosis of the following conditions:

Conditions

1. Diabetes insipidus
2. Acromegaly
3. Addison's disease
4. Hypoparathyroidism
5. Conn's syndrome

8.8 Genetic techniques

Options

a. Association studies
b. Electrophoresis
c. Linkage analysis
d. LOD score of Morton
e. Oligonucleotide probes
f. Mapping
g. Recombinant fraction
h. Recombinant hybridisation
i. Southern blotting
j. Twin studies

Lead in

Find one term each for the following statements:

Statements

1. The process of identifying the locus of a gene on the chromosomes by studying the extent to which it co-segregates with marker gene
2. Logarithm of the odds that the recombinant fraction has some given value divided by the odds that the value is 0.5
3. Comparison of different allele frequencies for a particular gene between disease population and a control population
4. A technique used to assemble correct DNA fragments from a gene library into a continuous overlapping stretch, which will contain the gene of interest
5. The number of recombinants in a family or group of families divided by the total number of offspring

8.9 MMSE

Options

a. Concentration
b. Constructional praxis
c. Delayed recall
d. Executive functions
e. Language – naming
f. Language – understanding
g. Long-term recall
h. Orientation in place
i. Verbal fluency
j. Writing

Lead in

Identify one cognitive process each that is tested by the following items in the Mini Mental State Examination:

Items

1. Spelling 'WORLD' backwards
2. Copying a diagram of interlocking pentagons
3. Carrying out a three-stage command
4. Repetition of three objects after a distraction task
5. Correctly stating current location

8.10 Neuroimaging

Options

a. Activation of primary auditory cortex on fMRI
b. Bilateral high signal in pulvinar nucleus of thalamus on MRI
c. Deep white matter hyperintensities on MRI
d. Diffuse cerebral oedema on CT
e. Focal atrophy of the frontal lobes on MRI
f. High signal lesions in cerebellar peduncles
g. Impaired dorsolateral prefrontal cortex function on fMRI
h. Medial temporal lobe atrophy on MRI
i. Multiple discrete white matter lesions with variable enhancement on MRI
j. Periventricular white matter changes on MRI

Lead in

Match each option each with the following conditions:

Conditions

1. Depression in the elderly
2. Auditory hallucinations in schizophrenia
3. Working memory tasks in schizophrenia
4. Variant Creutzfeldt–Jakob disease
5. Alzheimer's disease

8.11 Neuroimaging techniques

Options

a. Blood oxygenation levels provide a measure of regional cerebral blood flow
b. Can measure dynamic patterns of neurotransmitter binding
c. Good visualisation of white matter lesions
d. Inexpensive
e. Invented by Hans Berger
f. Invented in 1972
g. Resolution is poor
h. Uses a radioactive tracer to provide a measure of cerebral function
i. Uses non-ionising radiation
j. Utilises a process of spectroscopy

Lead in

Select two options each for the following techniques:

Techniques

1. MRI
2. SPECT
3. CT
4. fMRI
5. PET

8.16 Rating scales

Options

a. Akathisia rating scale
b. Anxiety rating scale and depression rating scale
c. Catatonia severity scale
d. Dementia rating scale
e. Depression rating scale
f. Extrapyramidal symptoms rating scale
g. Hypochondriasis rating scale
h. Mania rating scale
i. Negative symptom rating scale
j. Positive symptom rating scale

Lead in

Select one rating scale each to match the following names:

Names

1. Simpson–Angus
2. Young
3. Hamilton
4. Montgomery–Asberg
5. Barnes

8.17 Rating scales for children and adolescents

Options

a. BDI
b. CDRS-R
c. Connor's questionnaire
d. CY-BOCS
e. HoNOSCA
f. HDRS
g. K-SADS
h. MFQ
i. PSE
j. SDQ

Lead in

Select one rating scale each for use in the following situations:

Situations

1. Information from school about the severity of attention deficit hyperactivity disorder (ADHD) symptoms in school.
2. Clinician-rated severity of depression symptoms in a 14-year-old boy.
3. Information from school on symptoms covering a variety of psychiatric problems.
4. Ascertaining which psychiatric diagnoses are present in a comprehensive interview by a research assistant for the purposes of a research study of 13–17-year-old adolescents.
5. Severity of obsessive–compulsive disorder in a 13-year-old girl.

8.18 Rating scales in psychiatry

Options

a. BRPS
b. SANS
c. PSE
d. CATEGO
e. HRSD
f. SCQ
g. ADOS
h. HoNOS
i. HADS
j. SIS

Lead in

Match one instrument each with the following descriptions:

Descriptions

1. This interview retains the features of a clinical examination.
2. This is a computer program used to generate psychiatric diagnoses.
3. This instrument was developed to measure clinical outcomes in mental health.
4. This is a self-rating instrument.
5. This consists of standard activities that allow the observation of behaviour.

Answers

8.1 Choice of investigations

1-i. Studies from home movies (Green).
2-g. Studies of army conscripts.
3-a. Adoption studies.
4-h. Studies of cohorts of unmedicated patients.
5-d. Interventional studies.

8.2 Cognitive assessment

1-d. Executive frontal dysfunction (Jacoby & Oppenheimer-213).
2-a. Attention.
3-i. Semantic memory.
4-c. Episodic memory.
5-j. Working memory.

8.3 Cognitive function tests

1-e. Non-verbal intelligence (Lishman-94).
2-d. Memory.
3-b. Executive function.
4-h. Pre-morbid intelligence.
5-a. Brain damage.

8.4 EEG changes

1-g. Metabolic encephalopathy (NFP-73).
2-j. Typical absence seizure.
3-c. Focal structural lesion.
4-h. Myoclonic epilepsy.
5-a. Creutzfeldt–Jakob disease.

8.5 EEG waves

1-j. Theta waves (NFP-72).
2-a. Alpha waves (symmetrical, parieto-occipital).
3-c. Delta waves.
4-b. Beta waves (symmetrical frontal).
5-a. Alpha waves.

8.6 Endocrine investigations

1-b. Dexamethasone suppression test.
2-a. 24-hour urinary VMA.
3-j. Thyroid-stimulating hormone.
4-c. Fasting plasma glucose.
5-i. Thyroid antibodies.

8.7 Endocrine tests

1-e. Plasma and urine osmolality.
2-d. Oral glucose tolerance test with growth hormone levels.
3-h. Short ACTH stimulation test (Short Synacthen test).
4-g. Parathyroid hormone.
5-f. Plasma aldosterone and renin measurement.

8.8 Genetic techniques

1-c. Linkage analysis (OTP4-128).
2-d. LOD score of Morton (CPS7-160).
3-a. Association studies (OTP4-130).
4-f. Mapping (CPS7-159).
5-g. Recombinant fraction (CPS7-160).

8.9 MMSE

1-a. Concentration (NOTP-1628).
2-b. Constructional praxis.
3-f. Language – understanding.
4-c. Delayed recall.
5-h. Orientation in place.

8.10 Neuroimaging

1-c. Deep white matter hyperintensities on MRI (Rabins et al, 1991).
2-a. Activation of primary auditory cortex on fMRI (Dierks et al, 1999).
3-g. Impaired dorsolateral prefrontal cortex function on fMRI (Callicott et al, 2000).
4-b. Bilateral high signal in pulvinar nucleus of thalamus on MRI (CJD).
5-h. Medial temporal lobe atrophy on MRI (O'Brien & Barber, 2000).

8.11 Neuroimaging techniques

1-i,c. Uses non-ionising radiation; good visualisation of white matter lesions (O'Brien & Barber, 2000; Parsey & Mann, 2003).

2-g,h. Resolution is poor; uses a radioactive tracer to provide a measure of cerebral function.

3-d,f. Inexpensive; invented in 1972.

4i,a. Uses non-ionising radiation; blood oxygenation levels provide a measure of regional cerebral blood flow.

5-h,b. Uses a radioactive tracer to provide a measure of cerebral function; can measure dynamic patterns of neurotransmitter binding.

8.12 Neuropsychological assessment

1-d. Digit span.

2-k. Wisconsin Card Sorting Test.

3-j,h. Thematic Appercetion Test or Rorschach inkblot test.

4-f. Rey–Osterrieth Complex Figure test. An athematic perceptive, visuo-motor drawing task, which measures attentive analytical and perceptual–organisational skills, relative position of element to the whole and degree of precision. Distinguishes between mental retardation and brain damage. An alternative to Bender–Gestalt test.

5-g. Rivermead Behavioural Memory Test.

6-e. Minnesota Multiphasic Personality Inventory-2.

8.13 Neuropsychological tests

1-h. Test of visual memory, also known as the complex figure text.

2-j. Test of verbal memory, available for paired and unpaired words.

3-i. Test of visuospatial and perceptuomotor speed.

4-d. Test of intelligence, generally considered to be culture-free (CPS7-142).

5-f. Test of premorbid IQ.

8.14 Psychological tests

1-c. General health questionnaire.

2-a. 16 personality factor inventory.

3-f. Personality inventory.

4-e. Neuropsychological battery.

5-b. Adjustment inventory.

8.15 Psychometry

1-g. MMPI.

2-f. MADRS (CPS7-182).

3-j. WAIS (CPS7-142).

4-b. BPRS (CPS7-182).

5-h. MMSE (CPS7-142).

8.16 Rating scales

1-f. Extrapyramidal symptoms rating scale.
2-h. Mania rating scale.
3-b. Anxiety rating scale and depression rating scale.
4-e. Depression rating scale.
5-a. Akathisia rating scale.

8.17 Rating scales for children and adolescents

1-c. Connor's questionnaire. It is widely used to gain information from school on ADHD symptoms. There are also parent and adolescent versions.
2-b. CDRS-R (Children's Depression Rating Scale, Revised). It is derived from the HRSD.
3-j. SDQ (Strengths and Difficulties Questionnaire). It gives information on symptoms in emotional, hyperactivity, conduct, peer problems and prosocial domains.
4-g. K-SADS (Kiddie–Schedule for Affective Disorders and Schizophrenia). It is a paediatric version of the SADS.
5-d. CY-BOCS (Children's Yale–Brown Obsessive Compulsive Scale). It is the paediatric version of the Y-BOCS.

8.18 Rating scales in psychiatry

1-c. PSE (Present State Examination).
2-d. CATEGO – A computer program for processing data from the Schedules of Clinical Assessment in Neuropsychiatry.
3-h. HoNOS (Health of the Nation Outcome Scales).
4-i. HADS (Hospital Anxiety and Depression Scale).
5-g. ADOS (Autism Diagnostic Observation Schedule).

9. Psychological treatments

9.1 Brief psychotherapies

Options

a. Assertiveness skills
b. Core mindfulness skills
c. Dilemmas
d. Empathy
e. Narrative
f. Projective identification
g. Responses of others
h. Role transitions
i. Schema
j. Subjective units of distress scale

Lead in

Match one concept with each of the following brief psychotherapies:

Brief psychotherapies

1. Eye Movement Desensitisation Reprocessing therapy
2. Interpersonal psychotherapy
3. Cognitive analytic therapy
4. Core conflictual relationship theme
5. Dialectic behaviour therapy

9.2 Cognitive distortions

Options

a. Arbitrary inference
b. Automatic thoughts
c. Catastrophic thinking
d. Cognitive distortions
e. Dysfunctional beliefs
f. Emotional reasoning
g. Negative thoughts
h. Overgeneralisation
i. Personalisation
j. Selective abstraction

Lead in

The following are thoughts of a depressed person. Please select one term each for the thoughts:

Thoughts

1. "No-one likes me. Even when they say they want to help me get better, they don't mean it."
2. "My friend ignored me in the superstore. This means that everything that everyone tells me about how much they care is nonsense."
3. "If everyone does not like me, then there is no point in living."
4. "It rained when I went for a walk. Nothing works well for me."
5. "If I have a panic attack, I will lose all control and go crazy."

9.3 Couple therapy

Options

a. Behavioural couples' therapy
b. Behavioural-systems couple therapy
c. Brief dynamic therapy
d. Cognitive analytic therapy
e. Emotionally focused therapy
f. Milieu therapy
g. Psychodynamic therapy
h. Psychodynamic couple therapy
i. Structural therapy
j. Systemic therapy

Lead in

Find one term each to describe the interventions described below:

Interventions

1. Work based on the idea that the current problems in the family origi-nate in the past experiences of individual members, especially those of the parents.
2. Use reciprocity negotiating, communication training, structural moves, timetables and tasks, and paradox to solve problems couples encounter.
3. Try to help each partner to understand his or her own emotional needs and how they relate to those of the other person in the relationship.
4. The couple increases intimacy and improves their relationship by each assessing, acknowledging, and expressing their unmet feelings and needs.
5. An alcohol-dependent husband seen with his spouse to arrange a daily 'sobriety contract', in which the patient states his intent not to drink and the spouse expresses support for the patient's efforts to stay abstinent.

9.4 Dynamic psychotherapies

Options

a. Brief insight oriented
b. Cognitive–analytical
c. Interpersonal
d. Large group
e. Long-term dynamic
f. Small group
g. Supportive
h. Milieu
i. Client centred
j. Primal therapy

Lead in

Find one name each for the psychotherapies with the following features:

Features

1. Focuses on early experience and unconscious factors to explain abnormal thinking, emotions and behaviour. Lasts six to nine months.
2. Uses cognitive therapy techniques with a psychodynamic framework. Focus on interpersonal behaviour. A target problem list is made. Patient has an active role.
3. Lasts longer than nine months. Aims to increase the conscious recognition of the role of unconscious factors on current experience and behaviour by free association, analysis of counter-transference and interpretation.
4. Therapy, usually in a psychiatric hospital, that emphasises the provision of an environment and activities appropriate to the patient's emotional and interpersonal needs.
5. Emphasis is on the patient's self-discovery, interpretation, conflict resolution, and reorganisation of values and life approach, which are enabled by the non-directive, unconditionally accepting support of the therapist, who reflects and clarifies the patient's discoveries.

9.5   Family therapy

Options

a. Behavioural-systems couple therapy
b. Brief dynamic therapy
c. Cognitive analytic therapy
d. Eclectic therapy
e. Functional family therapy
f. Interpersonal therapy
g. Psychodynamic therapy
h. Functional family therapy
i. Structural family therapy
j. Systemic family therapy

Lead in

Find term each for the following family therapy interventions:

Family therapies

1. Focus on the present functioning of the family rather than the past experiences of the members
2. Focus on a set of unspoken rules that organise ways in which family members relate to one another
3. Focus on the present situation of the family and on how the members communicate with one another
4. Based on the idea that current problems in the family originate in the separate past experiences of its individual members, especially those of the parents
5. This therapy consists of a systematic and multiphase intervention map that provides a framework for clinical decisions, within which the therapist can adjust and adapt the goals of the phase to the individual needs of the family.

9.6 Features of psychological therapies

Options

a. Cognitive analytic therapy
b. Cognitive behavioural therapy
c. Counselling
d. Flooding
e. Group psychotherapy
f. Interpersonal psychotherapy
g. Psychoanalysis
h. Supportive psychotherapy
i. Systematic desensitisation
j. Therapeutic community

Lead in

Find one term each for the psychological treatments with the following features:

Features

1. Altruism, imitation, cohesion
2. Informality, group meetings, mutual help
3. Attention to provoking factors, homework assignments, highly structured sessions, monitoring progress
4. Exposure to highly anxiety-provoking situations until anxiety is diminished
5. Highly structured treatment with clear goals, suitable for bereavement, divorce

9.7   Features of psychotherapies

Options

a. Brief insight-oriented therapy
b. Cognitive–analytical therapy
c. Interpersonal psychotherapy
d. Large group therapy
e. Long-term dynamic therapy
f. Small group therapy
g. Supportive psychotherapy
h. Psychoanalysis
i. Transactional analysis
j. Group analytic therapy

Lead in

Find one term each for the psychotherapies with the following features:

Features

1. Focuses on early experience and unconscious factors to explain abnormal thinking, emotions and behaviour. Lasts six to nine months.
2. Uses cognitive therapy techniques with a psychodynamic framework. Focus on interpersonal behaviour. A target problem list is made. Patient has an active role.
3. Lasts longer than nine months. Aims to increase the conscious recognition of the role of unconscious factors on current experience and behaviour by free association, analysis of counter-transference and interpretation.
4. Goal is improvement in current interpersonal skills. It is done once a week for 12–16 weeks.
5. Lasts for three to five or more years. It is done four to five times per week for 50 minutes at a time. The patient is on the couch and the analyst is out of view.

9.8 Group psychotherapy

Options

a. ·Cohesiveness
b. Counter-dependency
c. Dependency
d. Free-floating discussion
e. Interpretation
f. Mirroring
g. Pairing
h. Role playing
i. Universality
j. Sociometry

Lead in

Select two concepts each for the following aspects of group psychotherapies:

Aspects

1. Reasons for the effectiveness of group psychotherapy
2. Factors in analytic group psychotherapy
3. Features that develop when people interact in groups
4. Basic psychodramatic techniques
5. Basic assumptions defined by Wilfred Bion

9.9   Group therapy

Options

a. Catharsis
b. Cohesiveness
c. Communalism
d. Dependency
e. Founded the Henderson Hospital
f. Mirror phenomena
g. Permissiveness
h. Pairing
i. Therapeutic community
j. Universality

Lead in

Choose the options associated with the following names:

Names

1. Bion (2)
2. Main (1)
3. Rapoport (2)
4. Yalom (3)
5. Foulkes (1)

9.10 Psychological therapies

Options

a. Cognitive analytic therapy
b. Contingency management
c. Exposure and response prevention
d. Flooding
e. Group psychotherapy
f. Interpersonal psychotherapy
g. Primal therapy
h. Psychotherapy
i. Systematic desensitisation
j. Therapeutic community

Lead in

Find one most appropriate term each for the psychological treatments with the following features:

Features

1. The patient is encouraged to enter situations that provoke unwanted behaviour and have previously been avoided. The patient refrains from carrying out the unwanted behaviour.
2. Therapeutic relationship, listening, emotional release, morale restoration, providing information, providing a rationale, advice, guidance, and suggestion.
3. Define and monitor behaviour, identify the stimuli and reinforcements, change the reinforcement, and monitor progress.
4. Make a hierarchy, learn to relax, enter the situation while trying to relax, and stay until anxiety subsides.
5. A therapy developed to effect a relief or 'cure' for neurosis that involves the patient learning to accept and allow his own feelings to surface by 'letting go' of conscious controls of the body and emotions, which then opens up the unconscious to awareness. The therapist only takes a supportive role.

9.11 Psychotherapeutic interventions

Options

a. Behavioural-systems couple therapy
b. Brief dynamic
c. Cognitive analytic
d. Eclectic family therapy
e. Non-directive play therapy
f. Milieu therapy
g. Psychodynamic family therapy
h. Structural family therapy
i. Systemic family therapy
j. Strategic family therapy

Lead in

Find one term each to describe the interventions below:

Interventions

1. Focus on the present functioning of the family rather than the past experience of the members. Established in Milan.
2. Focus on a set of unspoken rules that organise ways in which members relate to one another, including their established hierarchy. Minuchin developed this technique.
3. Focus on the present situation of the family and on how the members communicate with one another.
4. Based in the idea that current problems in the family originate in the separate past experiences of its individual members, especially those of the parents.
5. Focus on active interventions to fit specific problem areas in the family.

9.12 Psychotherapeutic options

Options

a. Aversion therapy
b. Biofeedback
c. Debriefing
d. Dialectic behaviour therapy (DBT)
e. Exposure and response prevention
f. Eye movement and desensitisation reprocessing (EMDR)
g. Implosion
h. Interpersonal therapy
i. Stress inoculation therapy
j. Systemic desensitisation

Lead in

Identify the treatment options that can be used in the following conditions:

Conditions

1. Simple phobia (2)
2. PTSD (3)
3. Obsessive–compulsive disorder (1)
4. Self-harming behaviour (1)
5. Bulimia nervosa (1)

9.13 Psychotherapies

Options

a. Cognitive analytic therapy
b. CBT
c. Counselling
d. Flooding
e. Group psychotherapy
f. Interpersonal psychotherapy
g. Psychoanalysis
h. Supportive psychotherapy
i. Systematic desensitisation
j. Therapeutic community

Lead in

Find one term each for the psychological treatments with the following features:

Features

1. Altruism, imitation, cohesion
2. Informality, group meetings, mutual help
3. Attention to provoking factors, homework assignments, highly structured sessions, monitoring progress
4. Exposure to highly anxiety-provoking situations until anxiety is diminished
5. Draws on the positive aspects of the therapist–patient relationship to maintain effective coping in patients

Answers

9.1 Brief psychotherapies

1-j. Subjective units of distress scale.
2-h. Role transitions.
3-c. Dilemmas.
4-g. Responses of others.
5-b. Core mindfulness skills.

9.2 Cognitive distortions

1-a. Arbitrary inference (OTP4-292; Secrets-211; CPS7-315).
2-h. Overgeneralisation.
3-e. Dysfunctional beliefs.
4-i. Personalisation.
5-c. Catastrophic thinking.

9.3 Couple therapy

1-g. Psychodynamic therapy (OTP4-754).
2-b. Behavioural-systems couple therapy.
3-h. Psychodynamic couple therapy.
4-e. Emotionally focused therapy.
5-a. Behavioural couples therapy.

9.4 Dynamic psychotherapies

1-a. Brief insight oriented (OTP4-744).
2-b. Cognitive–analytical.
3-e. Long-term dynamic.
4-h. Milieu.
5-i. Client centred.

9.5 Family therapy

1-j. Systemic family therapy (OTP4-757).
2-i. Structural family therapy.
3-d. Eclectic therapy.
4-g. Psychodynamic therapy.
5-e. Functional family therapy.

9.6 Features of psychological therapies

1-e. Group psychotherapy. The other curative factors in a group are universality, socialisation, interpersonal learning and recapitulation of the family group (OTP4-749).
2-j. Therapeutic community (OTP4-753).
3-b. Cognitive behavioural therapy (OTP4-732).
4-d. Flooding (OTP4-736).
5-f. Interpersonal therapy. Used in bereavement, social deficits, changes in roles, and role disputes (OTP4-732).

9.7 Features of psychotherapies

1-a. Brief insight-oriented therapy (OTP4-744).
2-b. Cognitive–analytical therapy (CPS7-320).
3-e. Long-term dynamic therapy.
4-c. Interpersonal psychotherapy.
5-h. Psychoanalysis.

9.8 Group psychotherapy

1-i,a. Universality, cohesiveness (Bion; Yalom).
2-d,e. Free-floating discussion, interpretation.
3-c,b. Dependency, counter-dependency.
4-h,f. Role playing, mirroring. The ten basic psychodramatic techniques are role playing, role reversal, interview in role reversal, soliloquy, aside, empty chair, mirror techniques, doubling, concretising and maximising, and future projection (Moreno, 1975).
5-g,c. Pairing, dependency.

9.9 Group therapy

1-h,d. Pairing, dependency. The other basic assumption is flight–fight (EPS-100).
2-i. Therapeutic community. Main coined the term (EPS-293).
3-g,c. Permissiveness, communalism. Other terms include democratisation and reality confrontation. Maxwell Jones founded the Henderson. Rapoport worked there (EPS-258).
4-j,a,b. Universality, catharsis, cohesiveness. Yalom's other nine therapeutic factors in group therapy are self-understanding, interpersonal input and output, existential factors, instillation of hope, altruism, family re-enactment, guidance and identification (EPS-258).
5-f. Mirror phenomena. Other group-specific therapeutic factors are socialisation and chain-condenser phenomena (EPS-301).

9.10 Psychological therapies

1-c. Exposure and response prevention (OTP4-736).
2-h. Psychotherapy.
3-b. Contingency management.
4-i. Systematic desensitisation.
5-g. Primal therapy.

9.11 Psychotherapeutic interventions

1-i. Systemic family therapy (OTP4-758; Bloch-240).
2-h. Structural family therapy.
3-d. Eclectic family therapy.
4-g. Psychodynamic family therapy.
5-j. Strategic family therapy.

9.12 Psychotherapeutic options

1-j,g. Systematic desensitisation, implosion, i.e. a type of flooding in vivo (behavioural methods are used; implosion or flooding is favoured less as it causes the most distress to the patient) (OTP4-736; DH).
2-f,i,j. EMDR, stress inoculation therapy, systematic desensitisation. The best evidence is for CBT but others can be used. Flooding can exacerbate some symptoms and therefore graded exposure is used instead. Routine debriefing is not recommended (OTP4-738; DH).
3-e. Exposure and response prevention – for obsessive rituals (OTP4-736).
4-d. DBT. Developed by Linehan. Used mostly in patients with borderline personality disorders. It uses a problem-solving approach (OTP4-739).
5-h. Interpersonal therapy (Hay & Bacaltchuk, 2004).

9.13 Psychotherapies

1-e. Group psychotherapy (OTP4-736).
2-j. Therapeutic community.
3-b. CBT.
4-d. Flooding.
5-h. Supportive psychotherapy.

10. General pharmacology

10.1 Agonists

Options

a. Serotonin$_{1A}$
b. Serotonin$_{2A}$
c. NMDA
d. Dopamine-2 receptor
e. Mu receptor
f. Sigma receptor
g. Omega-1 receptor
h. Serotonin$_3$
i. Muscarinic acetylcholine
j. Histamine$_1$

Lead in

Match the following agonists with one neurochemical system each:

Agonists

1. Zolpidem
2. Oxycodone
3. Fluvoxamine
4. Aripiprazole
5. Bromocriptine

10.2 Clinical pharmacodynamics

Options

a. 5-HT$_{1A}$ partial agonist
b. 5-HT$_{2A}$ receptor stimulation
c. Alpha-2 agonist
d. Buytrylcholinesterase inhibitor
e. GABA$_A$ agonist
f. GABA$_B$ agonist
g. MAO-$_A$ inhibitor
h. MAO-$_B$ inhibitor
i. NMDA receptor antagonist
j. NMDA subtype of glutamate receptor antagonist

Lead in

Select one mechanism of action each for the following drugs:

Drugs

1. Phencyclidine
2. Baclofen
3. Buspirone
4. Selegiline
5. Memantine

10.3 Drug dosing

Options

a. 5–10 mg/day
b. 6–10 mg/day
c. 6–12 mg/day
d. 10–20 mg/day
e. 15–30 mg/day
f. 40–50 mg/day
g. 80–160 mg/day
h. 150–600 mg/day
i. 300–900 mg/day
j. 900–1500 mg/day

Lead in

Select one best-fit adult dose for the drugs below:

Drugs

1. Donepezil
2. Reboxetine
3. Aripiprazole
4. Ziprasidone
5. Rivastigmine

10.4 Drug treatments

Options

a. Aripiprazole
b. Clomipramine
c. Diazepam
d. Haloperidol
e. Lithium
f. Lorazepam
g. Memantine
h. Rivastigmine
i. Sodium valproate
j. Thiamine

Lead in

Select one drug each for the following clinical situations:

Clinical situations

1. History of alcohol abuse and signs of sixth cranial nerve palsy
2. A mixed affective state induced by venlafaxine
3. Tourette's disorder with severe motor tics
4. Hepatic impairment and alcohol withdrawal
5. Cortical Lewy body disease with hallucinations

10.5 Enzymes

Options

a. Acetylcholinesterase
b. Alcohol dehydrogenase
c. Aldehyde dehydrogenase
d. Carbonic anhydrase
e. Catechol-O-methyltransferase
f. Choline-acetyl transferase
g. Cytochrome oxidase
h. Dopamine beta-hydroxylase
i. Monoamine oxidase
j. Tyrosine hydroxylase

Lead in

Match the actions below with one enzyme each:

Actions

1. It converts dopamine to norepinephrine.
2. Its inhibition is responsible for the effect of disulfiram.
3. It degrades monoamines in the synapse.
4. It degrades monoamines in the presynaptic neuron vesicles.
5. It degrades acetylcholine.

10.6 Half-life

Options

a. Aripiprazole
b. Atomoxetine
c. Carbamazepine
d. Chlorpromazine
e. Fluoxetine
f. Flupenthixol decanoate
g. Fluphenazine decanoate
h. Haloperidol decanoate
i. Quetiapine
j. Reboxetine

Lead in

Select one drug each to match the following half-lives:

Half-lives

1. Half-life of about three days
2. Half-life decreases during the first month of treatment
3. Active metabolite has a half-life of seven to nine days
4. Half-life of six to eight hours
5. Half-life of about 12 hours

10.7 Mechanism of action

Options

a. Buspirone
b. Clobazam
c. Duloxetine
d. Escitalopram
e. Moclobemide
f. Reboxetine
g. Ropinirole
h. Sildenafil
i. St John's wort
j. Verapamil

Lead in

Find one drug that matches each of the following mechanisms of action:

Mechanisms

1. Calcium channel blocker
2. Phosphodiesterase-5 inhibitor
3. Selective norepinephrine reuptake inhibitor
4. Inhibitor of norepinephrine and serotonin reuptake
5. 5-HT$_{1A}$ partial agonism

Answers

10.1 Agonists

1-g. Omega-1 receptor (GABA-A).
2-e. Mu receptor (opiate).
3-f. Sigma receptor (newly described).
4-a. Serotonin$_{1A}$ receptor (explains anxiolytic effects).
5-d. Dopamine-2 receptor (treatment of parkinsonism).

10.2 Clinical pharmacodynamics

1-j. NMDA subtype of glutamate receptor antagonist (OTP4-577).
2-f. GABA$_B$ agonist.
3-a. 5-HT$_{1A}$ partial agonist (OTP4-657).
4-h. MAO-$_B$ inhibitor (BNF47).
5-i. NMDA receptor antagonist (BNF47).

10.3 Drug dosing

1-a. 5–10 mg/day.
2-b. 6–10 mg/day.
3-e. 15–30 mg/day.
4-g. 80–160 mg/day.
5-c. 6–12 mg/day.

10.4 Drug treatments

1-j. Thiamine – for Wernicke's encephalopathy.
2-i. Sodium valproate – may be more effective than lithium.
3-d. Haloperidol.
4-f. Lorazepam – does not require hepatic metabolism, diazepam does.
5-h. Rivastigmine. Cholinomimetics are effective in the psychosis of LBD.

10.5 Enzymes

1-h. Dopamine beta-hydroxylase (CPS7-52.
2-c. Aldehyde dehydrogenase.
3-e. Catechol-O-methyltransferase.
4-i. Monoamine oxidase.
5-a. Acetylcholinesterase.

10.6 Half-life

1-a. Aripiprazole

2-c. Carbamazepine. The decrease in half-life is due to auto-induction of the cytochrome P450 3A4 enzyme involved in its metabolism.

3-e. Fluoxetine. The active metabolite is norfluoxetine.

4-i. Quetiapine. The drug is therefore administered twice daily.

5-j. Reboxetine. The drug is therefore administered twice daily.

10.7 Mechanism of action

1-j. Verapamil – treatment of mania and the prophylaxis of bipolar disorder.

2-h. Sildenafil – treatment of erectile dysfunction.

3-f. Reboxetine – antidepressant.

4-c. Duloxetine – a new dual-acting antidepressant.

5-a. Buspirone – anxiolytic.

10.8 Metabolism

1-j,c. MAO_B, COMT (EPP3-629; King-142; CTP7-44, 1138).

2-i,c. MAO_A, COMT.

3-i,b. MAO_A, Aldehyde dehydrogenase.

4-a. Acetyl cholinesterase.

5-g,j. Histamine methyltransferase; MAO_B.

10.9 New treatment indications

1-h. Topiramate. This drug has recently been shown to promote a decrease in alcohol intake and abstinence in ongoing drinkers.

2-i. Valproate.

3-g. Tetrabenazine. Possible adverse effects include depression and parkinsonian symptoms.

4-c. Lamotrigine, especially for Type II.

5-e. Sibutramine.

10.10 Pharmacodynamics

1-e. Buytrylcholinesterase inhibitor. Rivastigmine inhibits both acetylcholinesterase and butyrylcholinesterase.

2-g. $GABA_A$ agonist (OTP4-659).

3-l. Presynaptic alpha-2 agonist (OTP4-568).

4-b. $5-HT_2$ antagonist.

5-f. D_2 receptor partial agonist. The $5-HT_{1A}$ partial agonist and $5-HT_{2A}$ antagonist effects account for the lower incidence of sexual dysfunction.

6-l. Presynaptic alpha-2 agonist. Lofexidine causes less hypotension than clonidine (OTP4-568).

10.11 Precursors

1-c,a. Choline + Acetyl coenzyme A + Choline acetyl transferase, the catalyst → Ach (CPS7-49).

2-j,d,e. L-Tyrosine + Tyrosine hydroxylase → L-Dopa. L-Dopa + Aromatic L-amino acid decarboxylase →Dopamine. Dopamine + Dopamine B hydroxylase →NA. NA+ Phenylethanolamine N-methyltransferase → Adrenaline (CPS7-52; CTP7-44).

3-g. L-Tryptophan +Tryptophan hydroxylase →5-Hydroxy tryptophan. 5-HTP+ Amino acid decarboxylase →5-Hydroxytryptamine = Serotonin (CTP7-43; CPS7-57).

4-j,d. L-Tyrosine + Tyrosine hydroxylase → L-dopa. L-Dopa + Aromatic L-amino acid decarboxylase →Dopamine. (CPS7-54; CTP7-44).

5-f. Histidine + Histidine decarboxylase → Histamine (CTP7-45).

10.12 Receptors

1-g. High D2 receptor occupancy in striatum. PET scanning shows dopamine receptor blockade in the mesocortical dopamine system. The response to propranolol suggests adrenergic overactivity.

2-h. Low D2 receptor occupancy in striatum.

3-d. Dopamine receptor supersensitivity (OTP4-668).

4-j. 5-HT_3 receptor activation. There are fewer gastrointestinal side effects with mirtazapine due to 5-HT3 blockade.

5-i. 5-HT_2 receptor blockade. The ratio of 5-HT_{2A} to D_2 receptor affinities determines how much a drug behaves as an atypical antipsychotic. PET and SPET studies show that clozapine, olanzapine, risperidone and quetiapine a have high degree of 5-HT_{2A} receptor occupancy (> 90%) over their entire dose range. (Travis et al-1998).

6-b. Apolipoprotein E (OTP4-623).

10.13 Treatment indications

1-e. Lorazepam. Oral or parenteral benzodiazepines, e.g. lorazepam, is a first-line treatment for catatonia.

2-a. Clomipramine – has the largest effect size in obsessive–compulsive disorder.

3-d. Lamotrigine – is effective in bipolar depression and does not have a risk for manic switch.

4-i. Sildenafil.

5-j. Terazosin may reduce clozapine-induced hypersalivation.

11. Physical treatments

11.1 Acetylcholinesterase inhibitors

Option

a. 2–4 months
b. 6–12 months
c. 12 points
d. 18 points
e. Activities of daily living
f. Age of patient
g. Behaviour problems
h. Compliance
i. GP or specialist clinic
j. Specialist clinic

Lead in

Choose one item each that best fits with the statements below:

Statements

1. The National Institute of Clinical Excellence (NICE) guidelines suggest cholinesterase inhibitors may be prescribed in Alzheimer's disease for those with an MMSE score of more than ___.
2. The NICE guidelines suggest the diagnosis must be made in this/these clinical setting(s).
3. This is an important factor to consider when drug treatment is being considered.
4. Further assessments should be made after starting treatment within this time frame.
5. An assessment of this should occur before initiating treatment.

11.2 Antidementia drugs

Options

a. Donepezil
b. Galantamine
c. Insomnia
d. Memantine
e. Mild sedation
f. NSAIDs
g. Oestrogen
h. Paracetamol
i. Rivastigmine
j. Testosterone

Lead in

Please choose one option each that best fits the statements below:

Statements

1. This is a largely predictable side effect of cholinesterase inhibitors due to excessive cholinergic stimulation.
2. This cholinesterase inhibitor is metabolised at the site of action rather than by the cytochromes and hence has less potential for drug interactions.
3. This drug acts as an antagonist at the NMDA receptors.
4. Naturalistic case–control studies have suggested that elderly people who regularly take high doses of this agent often used in the treatment of arthritis have a reduced risk of developing Alzheimer's disease.
5. This sex hormone may have actions that may be preventive or disease modifying in Alzheimer's disease.

11.3 Choice of mood stabilisers

Options

a. Bendrofluazide
b. Carbamazepine
c. Captopril
d. Frusemide
e. Gabapentin
f. Lamotrigine
g. Lithium
h. Olanzapine
i. Sodium valproate
j. Topiramate

Lead in

You have a number of patients whose illnesses have been well controlled with mood stabilisers. However, there are some problems. Choose two drugs that you would consider:

Problems

1. A 30-year-old mother on lithium wants to breast-feed.
2. A 40-year-old man on lithium has been complaining of worsening psoriasis.
3. A 25-year-old woman stopped her lithium for a while and has now developed a rapid cycling BPAD.
4. A 50-year-old man on lithium has developed hypertension. His GP rang you to ask your opinion regarding the treatments to be avoided.
5. A young man's BPAD has been becoming increasingly uncontrolled with lithium alone. What will you add?

11.4 ECT in the elderly

Options

a. 1 per 10,000 patients
b. 1 per 100,000 patients
c. Cardiovascular
d. Cerebrovascular
e. Days or weeks around ECT
f. Little
g. Significant
h. Weeks or months leading up to ECT
i. Will
j. Will not

Lead in

Choose one option each that best fits the statements below:

Statements

1. There is ____ evidence that the cognitive effects of ECT are qualitatively different in older patients.
2. Most patients _____ have memory impairment post ECT.
3. _____ events are the leading cause of mortality from ECT.
4. Mortality from ECT is approximately _____.
5. Amnesia from ECT is usually for _____.

11.5 ECT mechanics

Options

a. Bilateral, suprathreshold ECT
b. Constant current, brief-pulse ECT
c. Constant voltage, sinusoidal wave ECT
d. D'Elia placement
e. Joules
f. Lancaster placement
g. Millicoulombs
h. Twice-weekly ECT
i. Unilateral, threshold ECT
j. Watts

Lead in

Choose one option each for the descriptions below:

Descriptions

1. An outmoded form of ECT
2. The most effective form of ECT
3. The least effective form of ECT
4. The unit used to measure the charge administered during ECT
5. The preferred electrode position for unilateral ECT

11.6 ECT practice

Options

a. Drug raises seizure threshold
b. Drug lowers seizure threshold
c. Drug increases seizure duration
d. Drug decreases seizure duration
e. Drug should ideally be discontinued prior to ECT
f. Medical condition is an absolute contraindication to ECT
g. Medical condition is a relative contraindication to ECT
h. An indication for ECT (as per the NICE guidelines)
i. Patient characteristics raise seizure threshold
j. Patient characteristics lower seizure threshold

Lead in

Find the options that apply to the scenarios below:

Scenarios

1. A 65-year-old man with a cardiac pacemaker presents in a catatonic state. He is not eating or drinking and is refusing medication. (2)
2. A patient with severe mania is not improving despite being on an adequate dose of sodium valproate. (3)
3. A 64-year-old man who takes NSAIDs for an arthritic neck has developed a peptic ulcer. He has been admitted to hospital as is severely depressed and suicidal. (3)
4. A patient who is anxious about ECT is requesting diazepam to help calm the nerves and to sleep the night before the treatment. (3)
5. A young afro-Caribbean woman with sickle-cell disease who developed neuroleptic malignant syndrome remains critically ill. (2)

11.7 Hypnotics

Options

a. Barbiturate
b. Benzodiazepine
c. Dibenzoxazepine
d. Imidazopyridine
e. Long half-life of parent drug >20 hours
f. Medium half-life of parent drug 6–20 hours
g. Medium-slow absorption
h. Pyrazolopyrimidine
i. Rapid absorption
j. Short half-life of parent drug <6 hours

Lead in

Identify three features each that relate to the following drugs:

Drugs

1. Flurazepam
2. Temazepam
3. Triazolam
4. Zaleplon
5. Zolpidem

11.8 Mood stabilisers

Options

a. Benzodiazepines
b. Carbamazepine
c. Gabapentin
d. Haloperidol
e. Lamotrigine
f. Lithium
g. Sodium valproate
h. SSRIs
i. Topiramate
j. Tricyclic antidepressants

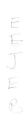

Lead in

Choose the most appropriate drugs for following cases of bipolar affective disorder:

Cases

1. A 42-year-old man presents with a severe depressive episode whilst on optimal long-term mood stabilisation.
2. A 23-year-old pregnant woman in her first trimester presents in a mixed state. She has never been on prophylactic treatment.
3. A 33-year-old woman, who had an episode of severe mania 18 months ago, now presents with depression with marked suicidal ideation. She was started on venlafaxine by her GP over the weekend.
4. A 35-year-old woman with liver disease has a history of four episodes of mania and two episodes of depression in the past year whilst on lithium.
5. A 37-year-old man has been on lithium for years. He still gets episodes of moderate depression where he is off work for several months at a time. He recalls being 'high' on two occasions many years ago. His GP suggested an additional mood stabiliser.

11.9 Pharmacodynamics of antidepressants

Options

a. Amitriptyline
b. Bupropion
c. Citalopram
d. Dothiepin
e. Duloxetine
f. Imipramine
g. Mirtazapine
h. Moclobemide
i. Selegiline
j. Venlafaxine

Lead in

Choose one option each to best fit the descriptions:

Descriptions

1. Preferential blockade of dopamine reuptake
2. Reversible inhibition of monoamine oxidase A
3. Blockade of alpha-2 adrenergic receptors
4. Irreversible inhibition of monoamine oxidase B
5. Blockade of reuptake of serotonin at low doses; of serotonin and noradrenaline at intermediate doses; and of serotonin, noradrenaline, and dopamine at high doses

11.10 Pharmacodynamics of SSRIs

Options

a. Blocks alpha-1 adrenergic receptors
b. Blocks calcium channels
c. Blocks sigma opiate receptors
d. Has anticholinergic action
e. No pharmacodynamic effect other than 5-HT reuptake inhibition
f. Stimulates 5-HT$_{2C}$ receptors
g. Stimulates the release of noradrenaline
h. Strong H1 receptor antagonism
i. Weakly blocks the synaptic reuptake of dopamine
j. Weakly stimulates NMDA receptors

Lead in

Match each drug with one option:

Drugs

1. Fluoxetine
2. Sertraline
3. Paroxetine
4. Fluvoxamine
5. Escitalopram

11.11 Switching antidepressants

Options

a. Cross-taper with caution
b. Discontinue over 4 weeks
c. Do not co-administer
d. May cause withdrawal symptoms, due to dependence
e. Stop drug immediately
f. Withdraw and wait 24 hours before starting new drug
g. Withdraw and wait 1 week before starting new drug
h. Withdraw and wait 2 weeks before starting new drug
i. Withdraw and wait 5 weeks before starting new drug
j. Withdraw then start new drug straightaway

Lead in

Choose the best options for the following scenarios:

Scenarios

1. A 64-year-old man experiences cardiac arrhythmias on amitriptyline. (1)

2. A 55-year-old woman who is being treated for depression and anxiety with venlafaxine continues to complain of insomnia. She has also developed dizzy spells due to postural hypotension. Therefore she is being changed to mirtazapine. (1)

3. A 25-year-old woman with atypical depression has not responded to fluoxetine and is now swapping over to moclobemide. (2)

4. A 34-year-old man lacking in energy and motivation was being treated unsuccessfully on citalopram and is now being changed over to reboxetine. (1)

5. A 28-year-old man with depression and anxiety is being switched over from tranylcypromine to paroxetine. (2)

11.12 Treatments for Alzheimer's disease

Options

a. Choline
b. Donepezil
c. Galantamine
d. Gingko biloba
e. Ginseng
f. Memantine
g. Nicergoline
h. Oestrogen
i. Piracetam
j. Rivastigmine

Lead in

Select one option for each feature below:

Features

1. An anticholinesterase drug, which also allosterically modulates nicotinic receptors
2. Half-life of 3 days
3. Inhibits both acetylcholinesterase and butyrylcholinesterase
4. Blocks NMDA receptors and potentially reduces excitotoxicity
5. Possibly reduces the risk of but does not treat Alzheimer's disease

Answers

11.1 Acetylcholinesterase inhibitors

1-c. 12 points (MPG7-234; NICE).
2-j. Specialist clinic.
3-h. Compliance.
4-a. 2–4 months.
5-e. Activities of daily living.

11.2 Antidementia drugs

1-c. Insomnia (MPG7-233; Katona & Livingston-83).
2-i. Rivastigmine.
3-d. Memantine.
4-f. NSAIDs.
5-g. Oestrogen.

11.3 Choice of mood stabilisers

1-b,i. Carbamazepine, sodium valproate (Bazire-209; CPS7-751).
2-i,b. Sodium valproate, carbamazepine (BNF47; MPG7-100).
3-i,b. Sodium valproate, carbamazepine (MPG7-107; OTP4-325).
4-a,c. Bendrafluazide and captopril (BNF47; OTP4-699). Avoid angiotensin-converting enzyme (ACE) inhibitors. Loop diuretics are safer than thiazides.
5-i,b. Sodium valproate and carbamazepine (MPG7-90; Bazire-29; BAP-B). Note: valproate is not licensed for long-term use.

11.4 ECT in the elderly

1-f. Little (Lawlor-231).
2-i. Will.
3-c. Cardiovascular.
4-a. 1 per 10,000 patients.
5-e. Days or weeks around ECT.

11.5 ECT mechanics

1-c. Constant voltage, sinusoidal wave ECT. This waveform delivers far more current than is actually necessary; the result is greater cognitive impairment without a corresponding increase in efficacy.

2-a. Bilateral, suprathreshold ECT. This is associated with the highest likelihood of response at the fastest possible rate.

3-i. Unilateral, threshold ECT. The response rate to this form of treatment is so low that ECT should probably never be administered thus.

4-g. Millicoulombs. Joules is the unit used to measure the energy delivered during ECT, while watts describes the power of the stimulus. ECT is conventionally dosed in millicoulombs of charge, although some devices still reckon the output in joules.

5-d. The D' Elia position. It maximises the interelectrode distance, thus minimising the shunting of current through scalp tissues from one electrode to the other. This electrode position also carries other advantages.

11.6 ECT practice

1-l,h. Patient characteristics raise the seizure threshold (male gender and older age); an indication for ECT (catatonia). A cardiac pacemaker is not a contraindication for ECT (NICE; ECT; MPG7-130).

2-h,a,d. An indication for ECT (severe mania); drug raises seizure threshold; drug decreases seizure duration (valproate).

3-i,g,h. Patient characteristics raise the seizure threshold (male gender and older age); medical condition is a relative contraindication to ECT (peptic ulcer, neck arthritis); an indication for ECT (severe depression).

4-a,d,e. Drug raises seizure threshold; drug decreases seizure duration; drug should ideally be discontinued prior to ECT (diazepam).

5-b,j. Patient characteristics lower the seizure threshold (young, girl). Sickle-cell disease is a relative contraindication for ECT. NMS is neither an indication, nor a contraindication for ECT.

11.7 Hypnotics

1-b,j,i. Benzodiazepine; short half-life of parent drug (6 hours); rapid absorption. The metabolite n-desalkylflurazepam has a long life (King-117, 135; Secrets-146; KSDT-67).

2-b,f,g. Benzodiazepine; medium half-life of parent drug (6–20 hours); medium-slow absorption.

3-b,j,i. Benzodiazepine; short half life of parent drug (6 hours), rapid absorption.

4-h,j,i. Pyrazolopyrimidine; short half life of parent drug (6 hours), rapid absorption.

5-d,j,i. Imidazopyridine; short half life of parent drug (6 hours), rapid absorption.

11.8 Mood stabilisers

1-h. SSRIs. SSRIs are less likely than TCAs to cause switching. Could try lamotrigine if antidepressants provoke mood instability (BAP-B).

2-d. Haloperidol. Treat mixed episode in the same way as mania. In pregnancy, use a typical antipsychotic rather than valproate, and avoid benzodiazepines (BAP-B; MPG7-100).

3-f. Lithium. Antidepressant monotherapy in bipolar disorder may precipitate mania. Use lithium for treatment and prophylaxis. Reduces risk of suicide (BAP-B).

4-b. Carbamazepine. Rapid-cycling disorder is unresponsive to lithium. Valproate is contraindicated in liver disease (MPG7-100).

5-e. Lamotrigine. It prevents depressions more effectively than manic episodes (BAP-B).

11.9 Pharmacodynamics of antidepressants

1-b. Bupropion. At higher doses, it may also inhibit noradrenaline reuptake.

2-h. Moclobemide.

3-g. Mirtazapine. Alpha-2 autoreceptor and heteroreceptor blockade releases noradrenaline and serotonin, respectively, from presynaptic neurons.

4-i. Selegiline. Hence, it is used to augment dopaminergic neurotransmission in Parkinson's disease. At higher doses (e.g. >20–30 mg/day), however, selegiline is an irreversible inhibitor of both MAO-A and MAO-B, making it similar to the classical MAOI.

5-j. Venlafaxine. Very approximate dose ranges for these three actions are probably <75 mg/day, 75–300 mg/day, and >300 mg/day, respectively.

11.10 Pharmacodynamics of SSRIs

1-f. Stimulates 5-HT$_{2C}$ receptors. Associated advantages are absence of weight gain, efficacy in bulimia, efficacy in bingeing and benefits in psychomotor retardation. Associated disadvantages are weight loss, anxiety, and agitation.

2-i. Weakly blocks the synaptic reuptake of dopamine. Advantages are absence of weight gain and benefits in psychomotor retardation. Disadvantages are weight loss, anxiety, and possible worsening in psychotic patients.

3-d. Has anticholinergic action. Advantages are less gastrointestinal adverse effects, less insomnia, and greater anxiolytic effects. Disadvantages are cognitive and somatic anticholinergic adverse effects and erectile dysfunction.

4-c. Blocks sigma opiate receptors. Advantages are decreased symptoms of anxiety and, possibly, psychosis. Disadvantages are increased gastrointestinal adverse effects.

5-e. No pharmacodynamic effects other than 5-HT reuptake inhibition. The advantage is that escitalopram carries the least risk of pharmacodynamic drug interactions amongst the SSRIs.

11.11 Switching antidepressants

1-e. Stop drug immediately, as this is a life-threatening side effect (MPG7-143).

2-a. Cross-taper with caution (MPG7-143; Bazire-187).

3-i,c. Withdraw fluoxetine and wait for 5 weeks before starting MAOI. Do not co-administer (MPG7-144; BNF47; King-175).

4-a. Cross-taper with caution. Can be used in combination in treatment-resistant cases (MPG7-144, 127).

5-h,c. Withdraw and wait for 2 weeks before starting new drug. Do not co-administer (MPG7-144; BNF47; King-175).

11.12 Treatments for Alzheimer's disease

1-c. Galantamine.

2-b. Donepezil.

3-j. Rivastigmine.

4-f. Memantine.

5-h. Oestrogen.

12. Adverse effects of drugs

12.1 Adverse effects

Options

a. Carbamazepine-induced agranulocytosis
b. Adverse reaction to lithium
c. Discontinuation syndrome
d. Hypernatraemia
e. Hyponatraemia
f. Lithium toxicity
g. Clozapine-induced myocarditis
h. Neuroleptic malignant syndrome
i. Serotonin syndrome
j. Torsade de pointes

Lead in

Match one cause each for the following scenarios:

Scenarios

1. A 65-year-old woman who has been on treatment for depression presents to the A&E department on a July afternoon complaining of nausea and dizziness. She gives a history of lethargy, weight loss, poor memory and cramps. She says she also takes 'water tablets'.
2. A 24-year-old male admitted 3 days previously with a severe acute psychotic episode has developed hyperpyrexia, muscular rigidity, profuse sweating and disorientation.
3. A 35-year-old woman has been on paroxetine for 2 years. Whilst on holidays she presented to the A&E with flu-like symptoms, insomnia, vivid dreams, irritability and tearfulness. She also describes "shock-like sensations" and dizziness exacerbated by movements.
4. A 40-year-old man with lithium-resistant bipolar affective disorder presents to the A&E with fever, a sore throat, a skin rash and mouth ulcers. The blood tests revealed low white blood cell (WBC) counts. He was started on another mood stabiliser recently.
5. A 35-year-old man who has been on clozapine for 2 months presents with repeated fainting episodes, chest pain, tachycardia, shortness of breath, increased temperature and leg swelling. His ECG shows ST segment and T-wave changes.

12.2 Adverse effects of antidepressants

Options

a. Amitriptyline
b. Fluoxetine
c. Mirtazapine
d. Moclobemide
e. Paroxetine
f. Nortriptyline
g. Phenelzine
h. Reboxetine
i. Trazodone
j. Venlafaxine

Lead in

Find one antidepressant drug each that has the following constellation of side effects:

Side effects

1. Weight gain +++; sedation ++; sexual dysfunction –
2. Weight gain +; sedation +; sexual dysfunction +++ GI symptoms ++
3. Weight gain +–; sedation ++; sexual dysfunction –
4. Weight gain +; sedation – –; sexual dysfunction +++; GI symptoms ++; Blood pressure changes+
5. Weight gain ++; sedation ++; sexual dysfunction ++; anticholinergic +++

12.3 Adverse effects of antipsychotics

Options

a. Akathisia
b. Carpo-pedal spasm
c. Cerebellar ataxia
d. Cholinergic rebound
e. Cogwheel rigidity
f. Dystonia
g. Intention tremor
h. Parkinsonism
i. Neuroleptic malignant syndrome
j. Tardive dyskinesia

Lead in

Select one option each for the clinical descriptions below:

Clinical descriptions

1. Rigidity, bradykinesia, cognitive impairment, tremor in a 55-year-old male who has been on chlorpromazine for over ten years.
2. Painful involuntary muscle spasms resulting in abnormal postures in a young male who received 10 mg of haloperidol IM for a first episode psychosis.
3. Pacing, shifting from foot to foot while standing and subjective restlessness in a middle-aged man who was admitted 3 weeks previously with psychotic depression and commenced on haloperidol in addition to increasing the paroxetine he had been on for a year.
4. Malaise, nausea, vomiting and diarrhoea in a man who was admitted 3 days earlier from a nursing home to an orthopaedic ward. All his usual medications were stopped on admission.
5. Involuntary repetitive movements of the orofacial and lingual region in an elderly female who has been on treatment for schizophrenia for 35 years.

12.8 Cardiovascular and endocrine side effects

Options

a. Aortic sclerosis
b. Aortic stenosis
c. Hyperprolactinaemia
d. Hypertension
e. Orthostatic hypotension
f. Pulmonary hypertension
g. QTc prolongation
h. Transient ischaemic attack
i. Ventricular
j. Weight gain

Lead in

Select one option each that best corresponds to the statement below:

Statements

1. Chlorpromazine is much more likely to cause this than amisulpride.
2. Concern over this has led to a restriction on the use of thioridazine.
3. Less likely to occur with clozapine or olanzapine therapy than with sulpiride.
4. Both clozapine and venlafaxine can cause this.
5. This is less likely with amisulpride than olanzapine.

12.9 Dermatological side effects

Options

a. Alopecia artefacta
b. Epidermolysis bullosa
c. Erythema multiforme
d. Flexural dermatitis
e. Hair loss
f. Hirsutism
g. Pigmentation
h. Premature ageing
i. Urticaria
j. Worsening of psoriasis

Lead in

Choose one adverse reaction each for the following drugs:

Drugs

1. Phenothiazines
2. Lithium
3. Imipramine
4. Mianserin
5. Sodium valproate

12.10 Drugs in pregnancy and breastfeeding

Options

a. Carbamazepine
b. Diazepam
c. Lithium
d. Paroxetine
e. Reboxetine
f. Risperidone
g. Sodium valproate
h. Sulpiride
i. Tryptophan
j. Venlafaxine

Lead in

Choose the drugs that best fit the following characteristics:

Characteristics

1. Teratogenic in pregnancy (4)
2. Moderate to low risk to prescribe to breast-feeding mothers (5)
3. Requires folic acid as a supplement during pregnancy (2)
4. Higher risk in breast-feeding (5)
5. Antidepressants with a high risk of causing discontinuation syndrome in the neonate (2)

12.11 Drug toxicity

Options

a. Confusion, headache, hypertensive crisis, seizures
b. Diarrhoea, vomiting, tremor, ataxia, seizures, coma
c. Diazepam to prevent seizures
d. Drowsiness, confusion ataxia, dysarthria
e. Flumazenil
f. Haemodialysis
g. Hypotension, hyperreflexia, QT prolongation, seizures, coma
h. Naloxone
i. Phentolamine
j. Pinpoint pupils, respiratory depression, coma

Lead in

For each drug below, choose one set of symptoms that indicate toxic levels and one treatment option. Use each option only once:

Drugs

1. Lithium
2. Methadone
3. Diazepam
4. Amitriptyline
5. Tranylcypromine in conjunction with mature cheeses

12.12   Dynamics of adverse effects

Options

a. 5HT$_{1A}$ autoreceptor
b. 5HT$_2$ receptor activation
c. H$_2$ receptor antagonism
d. 5HT$_{2A}$ receptor desensitisation
e. Alpha-1 adrenergic receptor blockade
f. D$_2$ antagonism
g. Decreased brain GABA function
h. H$_1$ receptor antagonism
i. M$_1$ receptor blockade
j. M$_3$ receptor blockade

Lead in

Select one option each to explain the following effects:

Effects

1. Tolerance to hallucinogens
2. Benzodiazepine withdrawal symptoms
3. Sedative action of trazodone
4. Postural hypotension with antipsychotics
5. Constipation, dry mouth with tricyclic antidepressants
6. Irregular menstrual periods with antipsychotics

12.13 Pharmacodynamics of adverse effects

Options

a. 5-HT$_{1A}$ receptor agonism
b. 5-HT$_2$ receptor agonism
c. 5-HT$_3$ receptor agonism
d. Alpha-1 receptor antagonism
e. Alpha-2 receptor antagonism
f. D$_2$ receptor blockade
g. GABA$_A$ receptor agonism
h. M$_1$ muscarinic receptor
i. H$_1$ receptor antagonism
j. H$_2$ receptor agonism

Lead in

Select one mechanism each for the following adverse effects:

Actions

1. Haloperidol-induced neuroleptic malignant syndrome
2. SSRI-induced anorgasmia
3. Trazodone-induced priapism
4. Mirtazapine-induced weight gain and sedation
5. SSRI-induced gastrointestinal disturbances

12.14   Side effects

Options

a. Carbamazepine
b. Clozapine
c. Gabapentin
d. Lithium
e. Mirtazapine
f. Selective serotonin reuptake inhibitors
g. Selegiline
h. Sildenafil
i. Short-acting benzodiazepines
j. Valproate

Lead in

Match each adverse effect with the best-fit drug options:

Adverse effects

1. Dose-dependent hair loss
2. Blue-tinged vision
3. Skin rash
4. Delayed or inhibited orgasm
5. Fine tremor

12.15 Side effects of drugs

Adverse effects

a. Agranulocytosis
b. Blurred vision
c. Dependence
d. Dysphagia
e. Hypersalivation
f. Insomnia
g. Nausea
h. Paraesthesia
i. Priapism
j. Urinary incontinence

Lead in

Select one most likely adverse effect each for the following drugs:

Drugs

1. Clozapine
2. Citalopram
3. Amitriptyline
4. Methylphenidate
5. Acamprosate

Answers

12.1 Adverse effects

1-e. Hyponatraemia. Antidepressants can cause hyponatraemia, possibly by SIADH secretion. Risk factors include old age, female sex, other drugs, medical conditions, and warm weather (MPG7-52).

2-h. Neuroleptic malignant syndrome (BNF47).

3-c. Discontinuation syndrome (Lishman-626).

4-a. Carbamazepine-induced agranulocytosis (1 in 20,000 risk).

5-g. Clozapine-induced myocarditis. One in 1300 risk in the first 6–8 weeks (OM4-316).

12.2 Adverse effects of antidepressants

1-c Mirtazapine (BNF47; MPG7-157; Bazire-186).

2-e. Paroxetine. Fluoxetine does not cause sedation.

3-i. Trazodone.

4-j. Venlafaxine.

5-a. Amitriptyline.

12.3 Adverse effects of antipsychotics

1-h. Parkinsonism (CPS7-267).

2-f. Dystonia.

3-a. Akathisia.

4-d. Cholinergic rebound.

5-j. Tardive dyskinesia.

12.4 Adverse effects of atypical antipsychotics

1-h. Prolactin elevation. The consequence can be amenorrhoea, infertility, breast tenderness, and related problems in females, and decreased libido in males.

2-b. Dry mouth and other anticholinergic effects.

3-i. QTc prolongation of 10 ms and longer; however, there is no evidence, to date, that there is an increased risk of torsades de pointes.

4-c. Hypersalivation. This may be treated with anticholinergic drugs and alpha-1 blockers such as terazosin.

5-e. Nausea, vomiting, and other gastrointestinal adverse effects. A possible reason is that aripiprazole is a $5-HT_{1A}$ receptor partial agonist.

12.5 Adverse effects of drugs

1-g. Skin rash. The risk of this adverse effect is reduced by slow upward dose titration.

2-j. Word-finding difficulty and other cognitive impairments. The risk is reduced by slow upward dose titration.

3-e. Nasal stuffiness is a temporary, dose-dependent side effect.

4-b. Bradycardia, due to increased peripheral cholinergic stimulation.

5-d. Impaired ability to read, due to pupillary dilation and impaired accommodation, resulting from the anticholinergic action.

12.6 Adverse effects of lithium

1-f. Greater than (CPS7-286).

2-g. Less than.

3-g. Less than.

4-b. Diarrhoea.

5-i. Seizures.

12.7 Adverse effects of psychotropic drugs

1-a. Amenorrhoea secondary to hyperprolactinaemia.

2-g. Stevens–Johnson syndrome.

3-h. SIADH can be caused by SSRIs.

4-d. Hair loss in 5%.

5-b. Cystic acne, usually a recrudescence of adolescent acne.

12.8 Cardiovascular and endocrine side effects

1-e. Orthostatic hypotension.

2-g. QTc prolongation.

3-c. Hyperprolactinaemia.

4-d. Hypertension.

5-j. Weight gain.

12.9 Dermatological side effects

1-g. Pigmentation (King-495).

2-j. Worsening of psoriasis.

3-i. Urticaria.

4-c. Erythema multiforme.

5-e. Hair loss.

12.10 Drugs in pregnancy and breastfeeding

1-c,g,a,b. Lithium – higher risk of Ebstein's anomaly; sodium valproate and carbamazepine – higher risk of neural tube defects; diazepam – higher risk of cleft palate (MPG7-206; King-119, 210, 353; Bazire-209).

2-h,i,d,a,g. Sulpiride, tryptophan, paroxetine, carbamazepine, and sodium valproate.

3-g,a. Sodium valproate, carbamazepine. Start folic acid 5 mg daily for at least a month prior to conception to help reduce the risk of neural tube defects.

4-f,b,j,e,c. Risperidone, diazepam, venlafaxine, reboxetine, and lithium.

5-j,d. Venlafaxine and paroxetine, because they have short half lives.

12.11 Drug toxicity

1-b,f. Diarrhoea, vomiting, tremor, ataxia, seizures, coma; haemodialysis (BNF47; KSDT-304).

2-j,h. Pinpoint pupils, respiratory depression, coma; naloxone.

3-d,e. Drowsiness, confusion ataxia, dysarthria; flumazenil.

4-g,c. Hypotension, hyperreflexia, QT prolongation, seizures, coma; diazepam to prevent seizures.

5-a,i. Confusion, headache, hypertensive crisis, seizures; phentolamine.

12.12 Dynamics of adverse effects

1-d. $5HT_{2A}$ receptor desensitisation/downregulation can cause tolerance to hallucinogens (Smith *et al* 1999).

2-g. Decreased brain GABA function (OTP4-561).

3-h. H_1 receptor antagonism.

4-e. Alpha-1 adrenergic receptor blockade (OTP4-669).

5-j. M_3 receptor blockade.

6-f. D_2 antagonism (OTP4-669).

12.13 Pharmacodynamics of adverse effects

1-f. D_2 receptor blockade (OTP4-670).

2-b. $5\text{-}HT_2$ receptor agonism. Also $5\text{-}HT_{1A}$ receptor antagonism. Nefazodone and Trazodone are $5\text{-}HT_2$ antagonists. Mirtazapine is $5\text{-}HT_2$ antagonist as well as $5\text{-}HT_{1A}$ agonist. Hence, they are less likely to cause anorgasmia.

3-d. Alpha-1 receptor antagonism (OTP4-692).

4-i. H_1 receptor antagonism.

5-c. $5\text{-}HT_3$ receptor stimulation by SSRIs. Mirtazapine causes $5\text{-}HT_3$ antagonism and hence no gastrointestinal side effects.

12.14 Side effects

1-j. Valproate.
2-h. Sildenafil.
3-a. Carbamazepine. Skin rash occurs in about 5% of patients. Stevens–Johnson syndrome is life threatening in some.
4-f. Selective serotonin reuptake inhibitors.
5-d. Lithium.

12.15 Side effects of drugs

1-e. Hypersalivation (BNF47).
2-g. Nausea.
3-b. Blurred vision.
4-f. Insomnia.
5-g. Nausea.

13.2 Management of affective disorders

Options

a. CBT
b. Citalopram
c. ECT
d. Lamotrigine
e. Light therapy
f. Lithium
g. Lorazepam
h. Olanzapine
i. Reassurance and education
j. Tryptophan

Lead in

Choose two treatments each for the following clinical presentations:

Presentations

1. A young woman with a history of dysthymia presents with a first episode of mild depression of 4 weeks' duration.
2. A middle-aged woman has failed to respond to an adequate trial of fluoxetine and has only partially responded to amitriptyline.
3. A middle-aged man with bipolar affective disorder presents with a relapse of mania. He stopped all his medications one year ago.
4. An elderly man with severe psychotic depression is now refusing to eat or drink.
5. A young woman complains of recurrent episodes of disabling hypersomnia, carbohydrate binging, lethargy and low mood occurring only in winter.

13.3 Management of anxiety disorders

Options

a. Alprazolam
b. Citalopram
c. Clomipramine
d. Gabapentin
e. Mirtazapine
f. Moclobemide
g. Phenelzine
h. Pregabalin
i. Risperidone
j. Venlafaxine

Lead in

Choose one British National Formulary (BNF)-recommended treatment each for the following conditions (use one option only once):

Conditions

1. Acute anxiety
2. Generalised anxiety disorder
3. Social phobia
4. Panic disorder
5. Obsessive–compulsive disorder

13.4 Management of schizophrenia

Options

a. Carbamazepine
b. Clozapine
c. CBT
d. Cognitive remediation therapy
e. Compliance therapy
f. Depot neuroleptics
g. ECT
h. Increase dose of current medication
i. Monoamine oxidase inhibitor
j. SSRI

Lead in

Identify one intervention each for the following scenarios:

Scenarios

1. A 20-year-old man with a history of hearing voices and persecutory delusions, partially controlled by risperidone 6 mg daily describes late insomnia, poor appetite and difficulty enjoying himself.

2. A woman with a ten-year history of schizophrenia has previously been treated with conventional oral neuroleptics, risperidone, and is now on 20 mg olanzapine. She no longer experiences hallucinations or delusions. Her self-care is poor and her affect is flat. She lives in a staffed hostel, is on disability living allowance and has few, if any, interests.

3. A 25-year-old man suffering from schizophrenia is admitted to hospital with his third relapse in 2 years. His key-worker thinks it is unlikely he takes his medication.

4. A 45-year-old man with a 15-year history of schizophrenia is experiencing troublesome hallucinations resistant to medication.

5. A 58-year-old woman, treated with clozapine, living in a staffed hostel, has few positive symptoms but her level of function, particularly social behaviour, is poor.

13.5 Prescribing in renal or hepatic impairment

Options

a. Chlorpromazine
b. Constipation
c. Diarrhoea
d. Haloperidol
e. Haloperidol and olanzapine
f. Hepatic
g. Lamotrigine
h. Lithium
i. Renal
j. Sulpiride and amisulpride

Lead in

Please find one option each for the statements below:

Statements

1. This mood stabiliser should be avoided in renal impairment
2. These antipsychotics are relatively safe in renal impairment
3. Sulpiride and amisulpride may be fairly safely used when this function is impaired
4. Drugs that cause this side effect may precipitate hepatic encephalopathy
5. This is the antipsychotic drug of choice in hepatic impairment

13.6 Prognosis of schizophrenia

Options

a. Acute onset
b. Daily cannabis use
c. Female gender
d. Good initial response to neuroleptics
e. History of schizophrenia in first-degree relative
f. Long duration of untreated psychosis
g. Male gender
h. Non-compliance
i. Positive response to placebo
j. Young age of onset

Lead in

Identify two factors, each linked to the following aspects of prognosis in schizophrenia:

Prognostic aspects

1. No clearly established relation to prognosis
2. Short-term poor prognosis
3. Short-term good prognosis
4. Long-term poor prognosis
5. Long-term good prognosis

13.7 Stages of change

Options

a. Action
b. Awareness
c. Contemplation
d. Early intervention
e. Maintenance
f. Motivation
g. Pre-contemplation
h. Ready for action
i. Relapse prevention
j. Understanding

Lead in

Identify the stages of behaviour change as per Prochaska and DiClemente:

Stages

1. Plans behaviour change, sets goals and assesses past successes and failures
2. Makes an initial attempt at modifying the problematic behaviour
3. Begins to realise that their behaviour has both costs and benefits and they are beginning to feel "two ways" about their behaviour
4. The final stage in the process of change
5. Content with one's behaviour and unlikely to express any need for change

13.8 Treatment of affective disorders

Options

a. Augmentation with thyroid hormone
b. Buspirone
c. CBT
d. ECT
e. Lithium
f. Lorazepam
g. Reassurance and education
h. Risperidone
i. Sertraline
j. Venlafaxine

Lead in

Choose treatment options for the following clinical presentations:

Presentations

1. A young woman with the first episode of depression of four weeks' duration (3)
2. A middle-aged woman with moderately severe depression that did not respond to amitriptyline, but showed a partial response to fluoxetine. Laboratory investigations showed subclinical hypothyroidism (1)
3. A middle-aged man with a diagnosis of bipolar affective disorder presenting with a relapse of hypomania. He had stopped all his medication a year ago (2)
4. An elderly man with severe depression with somatic syndrome (3)
5. A 38-year-old man presenting one week after losing his job. He was feeling low in mood, but is now starting to feel better as he has been getting other job offers (1)

13.9 Treatment of eating disorders

Options

a. CBT
b. Consider feeding against will
c. Diuretics
d. Family therapy
e. Gastric bypass
f. Fluoxetine 60 mg
g. Inpatient treatment
h. Oestrogen
i. Orlistat
j. Tricyclic antidepressant

Lead in

Choose the treatments for following cases:

Cases

1. A 20-year-old female with a body mass index (BMI) of 17.5 has a morbid fear of fatness and is restricting her diet. She has a transient low mood but no suicidal ideation. Her recent bone scan was normal. (1)

2. A 25-year-old woman with a past history of deliberate self-harm and substance misuse has become preoccupied with her weight. She indulges in episodes of uncontrolled excessive eating and then compensates for this by self-induced vomiting and use of laxatives. (2)

3. A 15-year-old girl with a BMI of 13 has been refusing food. She is now restricting her fluid intake as it makes her feel bloated. She has significant gastrointestinal and cardiac disturbance, potassium <2.5, and an abnormal bone scan. She is expressing suicidal intent. Her family is unsupportive. (4)

4. A 38-year-old man with high cholesterol and a BMI of 32 has reduced his weight by 5 kg in the past month by following his GP's dietary and exercise advice. (1)

5. A 22-year-old overweight girl has chronic low self-esteem issues but is not depressed. She often comfort eats up to 1300 calories at one time. (2)

13.10 Treatments for alcohol abuse

Options

a. Chlordiazepoxide
b. Chlormethiazole
c. Coronary artery disease
d. Diabetes mellitus
e. Intramuscular
f. Intravenous
g. Subtly lit
h. Vitamin B_6
i. Vitamin B_{12}
j. Well-lit

Lead in

Please find one option each that best fits the statements below:

Statements

1. Fewer adverse reactions are associated with thiamine given by this route
2. Nursing care in delirium tremens should be in this environment
3. Thiamine is also known as ___
4. This is a contraindication to disulfiram
5. This drug can have a dangerous interaction with alcohol

13.11 Treatments for substance misuse

Options

a. Acamprosate
b. Buprenorphine
c. Chlordiazepoxide
d. Disulfiram
e. Lofexidine
f. Methadone ampoules
g. Methadone liquid
h. Naloxone
i. Naltrexone
j. Urine drug screen

Lead in

Select one first-line treatment for the following clinical scenarios:

Scenarios

1. A 45-year-old man with alcohol dependence, hypertension and ischemic heart disease, has completed an inpatient detoxification and is motivated to stay 'dry'. He is requesting medication as an adjunct to counselling.
2. A 20-year-old man comes to the drug and alcohol clinic for the first time, stating that he has a 'habit' and injects heroin regularly. He wants to stop, but is worried about withdrawal symptoms.
3. A 22-year-old man with a history of heroin abuse was released from prison. He had not had heroin for several months. His girlfriend, who is on methadone, brought him to the A&E department. He is unconscious and has pinpoint pupils. She reports that he took only a small amount of her methadone.
4. A 28-year-old male addict has cut back to smoking 1–2 bags of heroin per day. He is requesting help to come off of it completely. He does not want an inpatient detox even though last time the detox failed because he became hypotensive. He is adamant that he does not want methadone.
5. A 31-year-old man has just completed a heroin detox and is requesting medication to help with relapse prevention.

Answers

13.1 Drugs for substance misuse

1-b. Buprenorphine. Partial agonist at mu receptor and antagonist at kappa receptor. Half-life >24 hours (Anderson & Reid-100; Core-440).

2-g. Lofexidine. Less likely than clonidine to cause hypotension. Reduces noradrenergic activity that underpins opiate withdrawal symptoms (Core-440).

3-j. Physeptone. Alternative name for methadone. Full agonist at mu receptor. Half-life >24 hours (Anderson & Reid-100; Core-439).

4-i. Naltrexone. Non-selective. Long acting. Half-life >72 hours (Anderson & Reid-98).

5-f. Disulfiram (Anderson & Reid-97; Core-431).

13.2 Management of affective disorders

1-b,a. Citalopram; CBT. Treat 'double depression' as a major depression (BAP-D).

2-f,a. Lithium augmentation; CBT. CBT has less evidence base (BAP-D).

3-h,f. Olanzapine for treatment; lithium for treatment and prophylaxis (BAP-B).

4-c,b. ECT; citalopram (NICE).

5-b,e. Citalopram; light therapy. Light therapy has limited evidence for effectiveness in Seasonal Affective Disorder. Treat major depression conventionally (CPS7-428).

13.3 Management of anxiety disorders

1-a. Alprazolam. For short-term relief of severe anxiety (BNF-47).

2-j. Venlafaxine.

3-f. Moclobemide.

4-b. Citalopram.

5-c. Clomipramine.

13.4 Management of schizophrenia

1-j. SSRI. (Hafner et al, 1999).

2-b. Clozapine. Clozapine is more efficacious than other antipsychotics, and may improve this patient's prominent negative symptoms. (Davies et al 2003).

3-e. Compliance therapy (Kemp et al 1998).

4-c. CBT (Kuipers et al 1997).

5-d. Cognitive remediation therapy (Wykes et al 2003).

13.5 Prescribing in renal or hepatic impairment

1-h. Lithium (MPG7-204).
2-e. Haloperidol and olanzapine.
3-f. Hepatic.
4-b. Constipation.
5-d. Haloperidol.

13.6 Prognosis of schizophrenia

1-e,j. History of schizophrenia in first-degree relative; young age at onset. Contrary to popular belief, long-term studies have not shown that early age of onset is predictive of poor outcome (NOTP-619).
2-b,h. Daily cannabis use; non-compliance.
3-d,i. Good initial response to neuroleptics; positive response to placebo.
4-g,f. Male gender; long duration of untreated psychosis.
5-a,c. Acute onset; female gender.

13.7 Stages of change

1-h. Ready for action (CPS7-373; Chick & Cantweel-159; Prochaska & DiClemente).
2-a. Action.
3-c. Contemplation.
4-e. Maintenance.
5-g. Pre-contemplation:

13.8 Treatment of affective disorders

1-i,j,c. Sertraline; venlafaxine; CBT.
2-a. Augmentation with thyroid hormone (CTP7-3065).
3-e,h. Lithium – for treatment and prophylaxis; risperidone can be used for treatment.
4-i,j,d. Sertraline; venlafaxine; ECT (CTP7-3063; NICE).
5-g. Reassurance and education.

13.9 Treatment of eating disorders

1-a. CBT. Her low weight may be causing her low mood, hence withhold antidepressants (NICE).

2-a,f. CBT; fluoxetine 60 mg. CBT or IPT for bulimia nervosa. A high-dose SSRI, e.g. fluoxetine may be used in addition or as an alternative).

3-d,a,g,b. Family therapy or CBT; inpatient treatment; consider feeding against will. Medication is not the primary treatment. Tricyclic antidepressants may cause cardiac arrhythmias. Oestrogen in adolescents may cause premature fusion of the epiphyses.

4-i. Orlistat. Only for adults with BMI >30, who have lost >2.5 kg, and other risk factors, e.g. high cholesterol, diabetes or high blood pressure (BNF47; NICE). Gastric bypass is the last resort and when BMI >40 (CTP7-1791).

5-a,f. CBT, fluoxetine 60 mg. Manage binge eating disorder similar to that of bulimia.

13.10 Treatments for alcohol abuse

1-e. Intramuscular.

2-j. Well-lit.

3-h. Vitamin B$_6$.

4-c. Coronary artery disease.

5-b. Chlormethiazole.

13.11 Treatments for substance misuse

1-a. Acamprosate. Disulfiram is contraindicated in coronary artery disease and hypertension. Naltrexone could be used but is less favoured (BNF47; Core-431).

2-j. Urine drug screen. Confirm dependency before prescribing (Core-440).

3-h. Naloxone for opiate overdose. The half-life of naloxone is 45 minutes, compared to methadone >24 hours, hence admit and observe overnight (Core-439).

4-b. Buprenorphine. Lofexidine can cause hypotension. Naltrexone precipitates intense but short-lived withdrawal and hence is used to 'kick start' detox. Requires symptomatic relief (BNF47; Core-440).

5-i. Naltrexone (BNF47; KSP9-455).

14. Developmental psychiatry

14.1 Aetiology in child and adolescent disorders

Options

a. Autism
b. Behaviourally inhibited temperament
c. Cannabis use
d. Enmeshment in family
e. Inconsistent boundary setting by parents
f. Increased cortisol levels
g. Living in the developed world
h. Maternal smoking in pregnancy
i. Parental tic disorder
j. Rise in oestrogen levels in female puberty

Lead in

Which of the above factors is most likely to be associated with the following clinical diagnoses in a 15-year-old girl?:

Diagnoses

1. ADHD
2. Depressive episode
3. Anorexia nervosa
4. Psychotic episode
5. Obsessive–compulsive disorder

14.2 Behavioural phenotypes

Options

a. Affectionate, clownish and easily amused
b. Compulsive and severe self-mutilation
c. Dementia-like picture in the fifth decade of life
d. Extraordinary verbal facility
e. Severe cold intolerance
f. Gaze aversion and social avoidance
g. Increased appetite and incessant skin picking
h. Learning disability and a schizophrenia-like psychosis
i. Preference for ball games over board games
j. Self-injurious and autistic behaviour

Lead in

Select one option each for the behavioural phenotypes of the following syndromes:

Syndromes

1. Fragile X syndrome
2. Prader–Willi syndrome
3. Cornelia De Lange syndrome
4. William's syndrome
5. Lesch–Nyhan syndrome

14.3 Child abuse

Options

a. 4%

b. 10%

c. 10–30%

d. Avoid exploring that issue but complete the interview before contacting Social Services

e. Explore in detail about the nature of possible sexual abuse

f. Keeping the family together

g. Parental consent overrides child's consent till age of 18 years

h. Safety of the child

i. She can consent to treatment if Gillick competent

j. Stop the interview at once and come out to call Social Services

Lead in

Choose one option each for the following situations:

Situations

1. A child aged 7 years discloses to you in your clinic that his uncle has recently been spending a lot of time with him and touches his private parts. What would you do?

2. The percentage of women perpetrating child sexual abuse.

3. The risk of further injury to children subjected to physical abuse.

4. In case of conflict of interests, the utmost importance is ___.

5. A 16-year-old girl presents to the A&E department with low mood and fleeting suicidal thoughts. She is diagnosed to have a major depression. She agrees for admission and treatment, however her parents say that she is just being difficult and insist that she is discharged.

14.4 Child and adolescent disorders

Options

a. Cluttering of speech
b. Delayed acquisition of speech
c. Displays repetitive behaviours
d. Equally common in boys and girls
e. Impaired concentration
f. Less common in boys than girls
g. Major violations of age-appropriate social norms
h. Marked dyspraxia
i. More common in boys than girls
j. Reduced eye-to-eye contact

Lead in

Match each condition below with the appropriate options:

Conditions

1. Specific reading disorder (2)
2. Childhood autism (4)
3. Asperger's syndrome (3)
4. Hyperkinetic disorder (2)
5. Conduct disorder (2)

14.5 Child psychiatric disorders

Options

a. 13–15 years
b. 15–19 years
c. Acute onset with rapid progression
d. Anger, somatic complaints and irritability
e. Chronic motor tic disorder
f. Gilles de la Tourette's syndrome
g. Gradual with social withdrawal and declining performance
h. Hopelessness, sleep and appetite disturbance
i. Non-organic enuresis
j. Normal child

Lead in

Match one most appropriate answer each for the following scenarios:

Scenarios

1. The parents of a 4-year-old child are concerned that the child passes urine involuntarily. There are no physical problems. The most likely diagnosis is ___
2. A recent increase in rate of suicide has been reported in males of age group
3. A 14-year-old with depression is more likely to present with complaints of ___
4. In childhood schizophrenia the course is often ___
5. A 15-year-old presenting with a 2-year history of only motor tics. The most likely diagnosis is ___

14.6 Child psychopharmacology

Options

a. Amitriptyline
b. Chlorpromazine
c. Clonidine
d. Dothiepin
e. Imipramine
f. Fluoxetine
g. Methylphenidate
h. Risperidone
i. Sertraline
j. None of the above

Lead in

Select on option each for the following situations:

Situations

1. An 11-year-old boy is brought to your clinic by his mother. He has no friends. Recently he tortured his cat and shows no remorse.
2. A 10-year-old adopted girl was brought by her mother with a history of being overactive and disorganised at home and at school. She was tried on imipramine by her GP for 3 months and there has been no improvement.
3. A woman brings her 16-year-old son to your clinic, saying that he is very anxious. He is unable to throw away anything and has been hoarding old magazines, notebooks and even shopping bags. He reveals that he has nonsense thoughts that come into his head. He recognises them as his own. He dislikes them, but can't get them out of his head.
4. A 14-year-old boy harms himself by cutting. He is very unhappy, has no appetite, can't sleep and hates himself.
5. A 15-year-old boy has struggled in his schoolwork for over a year, and has withdrawn from his friends. He reveals he has been hearing voices in the third person for two years, and believes he is receiving messages from the television.

14.7 Clinical genetics

Options

a. Angelman syndrome
b. Asperger's syndrome
c. Fragile X syndrome
d. Joubert syndrome
e. Lesch–Nyhan syndrome
f. Norfolk syndrome
g. Prader–Willi syndrome
h. Rett's syndrome
i. Turner's syndrome
j. Velocardiofacial syndrome

Lead in

Select one option each to match the following statements:

Statements

1. The most common contiguous gene syndrome, with a behavioral phenotype that includes learning disability and schizophrenia-like psychosis
2. The gene responsible is MECP2
3. Usually sporadic and associated with deletion on chromosome 15 of paternal origin
4. Monosomy (XO)
5. Associated with deletion on chromosome 15 of maternal origin.

14.8 Developmental syndromes

Options

a. Down's syndrome
b. Fragile X syndrome
c. Homocystinuria
d. Hurler's syndrome
e. Lawrence–Moon–Biedl syndrome
f. Lesch–Nyhan syndrome
g. Marfan's syndrome
h. Smith Magenis syndrome
i. Suffolk syndrome
j. Tuberose sclerosis

Lead in

Select one diagnosis each for the following clinical scenarios:

Scenarios

1. A 7-year-old boy was referred to the child development centre. He was pleasant and co-operative. He had a small mouth, small teeth and a high arched palate. His palpebral fissure was oblique and he had epicanthic folds. He had short, broad hands; incurved, little fingers; a single transverse palmar crease and hyperextensible joints.
2. An infant school pupil was referred with a history of delayed speech and language, not playing with other children and not paying attention in the class. His IQ was 60. Physical examination showed enlarged testes, large ears, long face and flat feet.
3. A 20-year-old female with epilepsy presented with white skin patches and subungal fibromata. A whole-body scan showed tumours in the kidneys, spleen and lungs.
4. A young male was referred to rule out Marfan's syndrome because of the skeletal features. He has mild learning disability. He also has ectopia lentis, fine and fair hair, and a history of thromboembolic episodes.
5. The ENT surgeon referred a 4-year-old boy with chronic otitis media to the developmental disability clinic. He has both conductive and sensorineural deafness, moderate learning disability, poor attention, overactivity, bruxism, stereotypical hand movements and self-injurious behaviour, including skin picking, biting and slapping.

14.9 Diagnosis in children and adolescents

Options

a. Asperger's syndrome
b. Attention deficit hyperactivity disorder
c. Childhood autism
d. Conduct disorder
e. Depressive episode
f. Manic episode
g. Oppositional defiant disorder
h. Rett's syndrome
i. de la Tourette's syndrome
j. Transient tic disorder

Lead in

Select one diagnosis each for the following presentations:

Presentations

1. A 13-year-old boy with irritability, initial insomnia, poor appetite, poor concentration, restlessness and reduced pleasure.
2. A 3-year-old girl with loss of previously acquired hand skills and speech, with hand-wringing stereotypies.
3. An 8-year-old boy with life-long difficulties in social interaction; rigidity, preoccupation with circumscribed interests; poor use of gesture, eye contact and other non-verbal communication; and monotonous, stilted speech. His first words came at 20 months, and he was speaking sentences at 30 months.
4. An 8-year-old boy who frequently ignores rules, is easily angered, initiates confrontations and arguments, and shows anger by frequently shouting at, but not hitting, adults and other children.
5. A 5-year-old boy with a 10-month history of motor tics (eye blinking, facial grimacing) and vocal tics (grunting, throat clearing and swearing).

14.10 Differential diagnosis in learning disability

Options

a. Asperger's syndrome
b. Dementia
c. Depressive episode
d. Fragile X syndrome
e. Obsessive–compulsive disorder
f. Panic disorder with agoraphobia
g. Panic disorder without agoraphobia
h. Psychosis (schizophrenia)
i. Rett's syndrome
j. William's syndrome

Lead in

Select one diagnosis each for the following clinical descriptions:

Clinical descriptions

1. An 18-year-old man has dysmorphic features and borderline intellectual functioning. Cognitive evaluation shows very good language abilities, but prominent deficits in visuo-motor integration.

2. A 42-year-old man with Down's syndrome presented with withdrawn behaviour, loss of confidence, forgetfulness, aggression and weight loss. Physical investigations including thyroid function are normal.

3. A 46-year-old man with Down's syndrome presented with withdrawn behaviour, loss of confidence, forgetfulness, aggression and weight loss. Laboratory investigations were normal. His symptoms gradually worsened despite adequate antidepressant treatment.

4. A 31-year-old man with borderline IQ is detained in a secure unit following a conviction for arson. He has a particular interest in lighters. He can describe in a formal, pedantic manner various 'lighter models', their manufacturers, their drawbacks, etc.

5. A 4-year-old girl's developmental milestones were normal until age 18 months. Thereafter she became progressively withdrawn, lost most of her developmental milestones, developed multiple hand-wringing movements and had a number of epileptic seizures and spells of hyperventilation followed by breath-holding.

14.11   Learning disabilities

Options

a. 1
b. 5
c. 15
d. 25
e. 35
f. 50
g. In females more than in males
h. In males more than in females
i. Only in females
j. Only in males

Lead in

Select one option each for the following statements:

Statements

1. As defined in ICD-10, the cut-off between mild and moderate mental retardation is an IQ of ___.
2. Prader–Willi syndrome is associated with a deletion on chromosome number ___.
3. The population prevalence of autism is approximately ___ per 10,000.
4. Rett's syndrome occurs ___.
5. Fragile X occurs ___.

14.12 Pharmacology in children

Options

a. Amitriptyline
b. Clomipramine
c. Clonidine
d. Fluoxetine
e. Imipramine
f. Methylphenidate
g. Olanzapine
h. Risperidone
i. Venlafaxine
j. None of the above

Lead in

Choose one drug each for the following scenarios:

Scenarios

1. A 14-year-old boy comes to your clinic with his parents, complaining of feeling ashamed and embarrassed. He admits that he swears and grunts in public and at times makes inappropriate obscene gestures, even if he does not mean to. He has had involuntary, jerky movements of his arms and face on and off for the last 2 years.

2. The parents of a 10-year-old girl bring her to your clinic complaining that she spends a lot of time in the bathroom. She admits to having some "silly thoughts" that come to her mind that she hates and the only way she can avoid them is by bathing and dressing in a "particular way".

3. You see a 7-year-old boy in your clinic with his mother. He has been attending the child behaviour group for some time with no progress. The main complaints are restlessness, overactivity, poor concentration and impatience.

4. The parents of a 10-year-old boy with autism and attending a special school bring him to your clinic, as they are unable to manage his aggression at home and difficult behaviour.

5. An 8-year-old girl has been receiving treatment for ADHD. Her parents are concerned that of late she makes some funny, jerky movements in her arms. She also grimaces.

14.13 School non-attendance

Options

a. Agoraphobia
b. Asperger's syndrome
c. Autism
d. Conduct disorder
e. Depressive episode
f. Obsessive–compulsive disorder
g. Oppositional defiant disorder
h. Panic disorder
i. Separation anxicty disorder
j. Social phobia

Lead in

Select one diagnosis each for school non-attendance for the following reasons:

Reasons

1. Previously sociable and did well at school. Now can't see the point in going to school or seeing friends
2. Does not like being in public places, such as the school, shops and buses
3. Worries that something bad may happen to his mother when he is at school
4. Would rather spend the day out with friends in the shopping centre, sometimes shoplifting or joyriding
5. Initially found it hard to cope with primary school, but with help adjusted to it and liked the routine, providing his teacher was not absent, and scored above-average marks in all subjects. Found the transition to secondary school very difficult, in particular the large number of new people and having to cope with moving around from class to class.

14.14 Treatment in children and adolescents

Options

a. Appropriate educational provision
b. Cognitive-behavioural family-based therapy
c. Haloperidol
d. Imipramine
e. Interpersonal therapy
f. Lithium
g. Multisystemic therapy
h. Paroxetine
i. Psychodynamic psychotherapy
j. Systemic family therapy

Lead in

Select one treatment each for the following disorders if found in a 15-year-old boy:

Diagnoses

1. Obsessive–compulsive disorder
2. Depressive episode
3. Hyperkinetic disorder
4. Autism
5. Conduct disorder

Answers

14.1 Aetiology in child and adolescent disorders

1-h. Maternal smoking in pregnancy – increases the risk of ADHD and conduct disorder. Inconsistent boundary setting does not itself cause ADHD, but makes behavioural problems more likely in ADHD (Rutter & Taylor-406).

2-f. Increased cortisol levels – are associated with adolescent depression and also with increased risk of the onset of depression in adolescents at risk for depression (Goodyer *et al* 1996).

3-g. Living in the developed world. Anorexia nervosa is found much more widely in the developed than developing world, suggesting an important role for western social ideals of thinness. There is no evidence for the role of the 'anorexigenic' family background (Goodman & Scott-151).

4-c. Cannabis use – can both cause an acute psychotic episode and increase the risk for a later psychotic disorder (Arseneault *et al* 2004).

5-i. Parental tic disorder. There is significant overlap between OCD and tic disorder, both within individuals and within families (Rutter & Taylor-579).

14.2 Behavioural phenotypes

1-f. Gaze aversion and social avoidance (Fraser & Kerr-86, 94).
2-g. Incessant skin picking.
3-j. Self-injurious and autistic behaviour.
4-d. Extraordinary verbal facility.
5-b. Compulsive and severe self-mutilation.

14.3 Child abuse

1-d. Avoid exploring that issue but complete the interview before contacting Social Services. Exploring the issues of abuse on your own can mislead the child and alter evidence. However, stopping the interview abruptly will be traumatic to the child.

2-b. 10% (OTP4-859).
3-c. 10–30% (OTP4-857).
4-h. Safety of the child.
5-i. She can consent to treatment if Gillick competent. Though parents give consent on behalf of children up to the age of 18 years, children aged between 16 and 18 years can give consent to their own treatment if Gillick competent.

14.4 Child and adolescent disorders

1-b,i. Delayed acquisition of speech; more common in boys than girls.

2-j,b,i,c. Reduced eye-to-eye contact; delayed acquisition of speech; more common in boys than girls; displays repetitive behaviours.

3-i,c,j. More common in boys than girls; displays repetitive behaviours; reduced eye-to-eye contact.

4-i,e. More common in boys than girls; impaired concentration.

5-g,i. Major violations of age-appropriate social norms. More common in boys than girls.

14.5 Child psychiatric disorders

1-j. Normal child. Non-organic enuresis is diagnosed only after the age of 5 years (ICD-10).

2-b. 15–19 years (OTP4-514).

3-d. Anger, somatic complaints and irritability. In adolescents, hopelessness and altered sleep and appetite are less common than irritability, anger and somatic complaints (OTP4-853; CPS7-604).

4-g. Gradual with social withdrawal and declining performance (OTP4-853).

5-e. Chronic motor tic disorder. A diagnosis of Tourette's disorder requires both motor and vocal tics at some time during the illness (ICD-10).

14.6 Child psychopharmacology

1-j. None of the above. Pharmacotherapy is not usually used in conduct disorder (Goodman & Scott).

2-g. Methylphenidate for ADHD.

3-i. Sertraline. Although now contraindicated for treatment in depression in patients aged below 18 years, sertraline is licensed in the UK for the treatment of childhood OCD (MHRA). Fluoxetine is not licensed in the UK for treatment of any condition in under 18s (BNF47).

4-f. Fluoxetine. Not licensed in the UK for treatment of depression in children, but licensed in the USA. Fluoxetine has the best evidence base for treatment of depression in children.

5-h. Risperidone.

14.7 Clinical genetics

1-j. Velocardiofacial syndrome (Fraser & Kerr-54, 76).

2-h. Rett's syndrome.

3-g. Prader–Willi syndrome.

4-i. Turner's syndrome.

5-a. Angelman syndrome.

14.8 Developmental syndromes

1-a. Down's syndrome (OTP4-881; Fraser & Kerr-92).
2-b. Fragile X syndrome.
3-j. Tuberous sclerosis.
4-c. Homocystinuria.
5-h. Smith Magenis syndrome.

14.9 Diagnosis in children and adolescents

1-e. Depressive episode. DSM-IV but not ICD-10 allows irritability as the presenting mood symptom for diagnosis of depression in childhood and adolescence. The anhedonia makes depression a more appropriate diagnosis than mania (DSM-IV).
2-h. Rett's syndrome (ICD-10).
3-a. Asperger's syndrome. It is similar to autism except that language development is not delayed. However, there can still be qualitative abnormalities in language, such as monotony, and in non-verbal communication (ICD-10).
4-g. Oppositional defiant disorder. It is characterised by persistently deviant and disobedient behaviour, often with a lot of anger. It is differentiated from conduct disorder by the absence of behaviour that violates the law and basic rights of others, such as assault and theft (ICD-10).
5-j. Transient tic disorder. It is differentiated from other tic disorders by duration of less than 12 months (ICD-10; DSM-IV).

14.10 Differential diagnosis in learning disability

1-j. William's syndrome (Fraser & Kerr-91).
2-c. Depressive episode.
3-b. Dementia.
4-a. Asperger's syndrome.
5-i. Rett's syndrome.

14.11 Learning disability

1-f. 50 (Fraser & Kerr).
2-c. 15.
3-b. 5.
4-i. Only in females.
5-h. In males more than in females.

14.12 Pharmacology in children

1-h,c. Risperidone or clonidine for Tourette's disorder (MPG7-169).
2-d. Fluoxetine. Clomipramine is a second-line drug for OCD.
3-f. Methylphenidate or dexamphetamine for ADHD.
4-h. Risperidone. Risperidone is effective in managing aggression, difficult behaviour and hyperactivity in children with autism.
5-c Clonidine. It is an unlicensed second-line drug in ADHD. It may improve the tics caused by stimulant drugs.

14.13 School non-attendance

1-e. Depressive episode. If school non-attendance is due to poor motivation, especially if this is global for all activities, depression should be considered.

2-a. Agoraphobia. A significant cause for anxiety around going to school is when agoraphobia is causing a general anxiety around being out in public places.

3-i. Separation anxiety disorder. It is important to find out whether anxiety about school is due to anxiety about *being at school* or anxiety about *being away from home* (as in separation anxiety).

4-d. Conduct disorder (CD). Truancy is one of the symptoms of CD. The acts of theft clearly distinguish CD from ODD.

5-b. Asperger's syndrome. It is much harder for children with autistic spectrum disorders to adjust to secondary school with different teachers and classrooms for each lesson, and all the new people, than to primary school with the same class, teacher and pupils for each lesson. Most children with autism have an IQ below 100, and hence the diagnosis is likely to be Asperger's syndrome rather than autism.

14.14 Treatment in children and adolescents

1-b. Cognitive-behavioural family-based therapy. Actively engage families in order to ensure that they are not involved in the rituals of the child and that they positively reinforce non-OCD activities. Clomipramine, fluoxetine, fluvoxamine and sertraline are effective in OCD in children and have a positive benefit:risk balance. (McClellan & Werry, 2003; Barrett *et al*, 2004; MHRA).

2-e. Interpersonal therapy. IPT and individual CBT are effective in adolescent depression. Fluoxetine has a proven positive benefit:risk balance for adolescents (Mufson *et al*, 1999).

3-d. Imipramine. While methylphenidate and dexamphetamine are the first-line medical treatment for HKD/ADHD, second-line treatments include TCAs and clonidine.

4-a. Appropriate educational provision. The key interventions in autism are social, in particular education, and support for parents. Haloperidol and risperidone reduce some of the symptoms of autism, but the side effects limit the benefit:harm balance, especially if seen from the patient's perspective.

5-g. Multisystemic therapy. It is the most cost-effective treatment for adolescent conduct disorder. Family therapy has limited efficacy in adolescents, although it can be very effective in younger children. Antipsychotic drugs reduce aggression, but the side effects and poor compliance limit their use.

15. Statistics and research methodolgy

15.1 Alternatives to standard statistical procedures

Options

a. Fisher's exact test
b. Kendell's tau
c. Kolmogorov–Smirnov test
d. Kruskall–Wallis test
e. Mann–Whitney test
f. Spearman's test
g. Student–Neuman–Keuls test
h. Survival analysis
i. Tukey's test
j. Wilcoxon signed-rank tests

Lead in

All statistical procedures require certain assumptions to be fulfilled before they are applied. If these assumptions are not fulfilled, we chose alternative tests. Find one such alternative each for the following tests:

Tests

1. Independent sample *t*-test
2. Paired *t*-test
3. One-way analysis of variance
4. Pearson's product moment correlation
5. Chi square test

15.2 Biases

Options

a. Attrition bias
b. Berkson's bias
c. Confounding bias
d. Information bias
e. Membership bias
f. Neyman's bias
g. Publication bias
h. Recall bias
i. Selection bias
j. Unmasking bias

Lead in

Identify one type of bias each in the following situations:

Situations

1. In a case–control study looking at the association between the use of antihypertensive medication and depression, subjects with depression may be more likely to remember what medication they have had, due to the potential importance of this issue to them.
2. In a cohort study looking at the long-term association between cannabis use and schizophrenia, subjects in the cannabis group were more likely to drop out of follow-up.
3. A case–control study investigating the association between poor social support and depression recruits depressed subjects from psychiatric hospital in-patients.
4. In the testing of a screening tool for depression, the same psychiatrist applies the screening tool as carries out the diagnostic assessment.
5. In a placebo-controlled trial for a new antidepressant, group allocation is based on hospital numbers, so the psychiatrist who enters patients for the study knows in advance which treatment group they will be in.

15.3 Characteristics of a good test

Options

a. Coherence
b. Negative predictive value
c. Normal distribution
d. Positive predictive value
e. Reliability
f. Sensitivity
g. Specificity
h. Standardisation
i. Symmetry
j. Validity

Lead in

Match each description below with one term above:

Descriptions

1. Removing weaknesses from a test and making it appropriate to a population
2. Ability of a test to identify a case
3. Replicability of a test
4. Ability of a test to identify non-cases
5. Ability of a test to tap a true construct

15.4 Multivariate statistical procedures

Options

a. Analysis of covariance
b. Cluster analysis
c. Factor analysis
d. Kaplan–Meier survival analysis
e. Logistic regression analysis
f. Multiple regression analysis
g. Multivariate analysis of variance (MANOVA)
h. Path analysis
i. Probit analysis
j. Repeated measures multivariate analysis of variance (RMANOVA)

Lead in

Choose one statistical test each that fits the following descriptions:

Descriptions

1. Simultaneously compares several independent means across groups
2. Compares the means of the same variable obtained from one or more groups at different points in time
3. Predicts the value of a quantitative dependent variable based on the values of several independent variables
4. Predicts the value of a dichotomous variable based on the values of several independent variables
5. Reduces a large number of variables into a smaller group of representative variables

15.5 Statistical concepts

Options

a. Concurrent validity
b. Construct validity
c. Convergent and divergent validity
d. Criterion validity
e. Historical validity
f. Internal reliability
g. Inter-rater and intra-rater reliability
h. Known group validity
i. Predictive validity
j. Retrospective validity

Lead in

Select one option each for the descriptions below:

Descriptions

1. Assesses the extent to which a new measure can predict future variables
2. Can be assessed where no established 'gold standard' external criterion exists
3. Is tested by comparing measures obtained with the new instrument to those obtained with an existing 'gold standard' measure
4. Is tested by the extent to which the new measure relates to other measures taken at the same time
5. These measures should be tested in relation to each other

15.6 Statistical tests

Options

a. ANCOVA
b. ANOVA
c. Chi-squared
d. Fisher's exact test
e. Kruskal–Wallis test
f. Mann–Whitney test
g. Multiple linear regression
h. Multiple logistic regression
i. Pearson
j. Student's *t*-test

Lead in

Select one statistical test each for the following situations:

Situations

1. Investigation of the association between multiple risk factors and the risk of developing schizophrenia
2. Comparison of the risk of developing schizophrenia in two groups of 1000 people – one of people who have used cannabis and one of people who have never used cannabis.
3. Comparison of final outcome measures between the three groups (CBT, SSRI, and placebo) in a depression treatment study. Results are normally distributed.
4. Comparison of a measure of coping styles in a depressed and a control group. Results have skewed distributions, despite transformation.
5. Comparison of final outcome measures between two groups (placebo and antipsychotic) in a psychosis treatment study. Despite random allocation to groups, there was a significant baseline difference between groups. Results are normally distributed.

15.7 Study designs

Options

a. Case–control study
b. Cost–benefit study
c. Cost-effectiveness study
d. Cost utility study
e. Double-blind randomised, controlled trial
f. Ecological study
g. Open-label randomised controlled study
h. Patient preference controlled study
i. Prospective cohort study
j. Retrospective cohort study

Lead in

Select one term each for the following studies:

Studies

1. Comparison of costs per QALY between two different treatments
2. Rates of MMR vaccination and number of new cases of autism over the next three years are measured in all regions of a country. Vaccination rates and autism incidence are then compared between regions.
3. A group of subjects born 40 years ago is found from birth registers. Presence or absence of obstetric complications is ascertained from the notes. Subjects and relatives are then interviewed and medical records examined to look for the presence or absence of schizophrenia.
4. In a treatment study comparing a new experimental type of hormone treatment for depression, subjects are randomised to receiving the hormone or an SSRI. For ethical reasons, patients and investigators know what treatment arm subjects are in.
5. In an RCT comparing two models of service delivery for patients with schizophrenia, all costs and treatment outcomes are compared for the two groups. A new treatment is more expensive but leads to better clinical outcomes.

15.8 Treatment effects

Options

a. Absolute benefit increase
b. Absolute risk reduction
c. Likelihood ratio
d. Negative predictive value
e. Number needed to treat
f. Odds ratio
g. Positive predictive value
h. Relative benefit increase
i. Relative risk
j. Relative risk reduction

Lead in

Match one term each for the following equations:

Equations

1. Experimental event rate (EER)–Control event rate (CER)
2. Experimental event rate (EER)/Control event rate (CER)
3. CER–EER
4. CER–EER/CER
5. 1/EER–CER

15.9 Univariate statistics

Options

a. ANOVA
b. Chi-square test
c. Covariance matrix
d. Kappa coefficient
e. Kolmogorov–Smirnov tests
f. Kruskall–Wallis test
g. Levine's test
h. Mann–Whitney test
i. Pearson's product-moment correlation coefficient
j. Student's *t*-test

Lead in

Choose one test each for the following purposes:

Purposes

1. Compare the means of two groups
2. Compare the means of two or more groups
3. Assess the strength of association between two quantitative variables
4. Compare proportions between two or more groups.
5. Measure reliability

15.10 Validity

Options

a. Criterion validity
b. Convergent validity
c. Content validity
d. Construct validity
e. Divergent validity
f. Face validity
g. Inter-rater reliability
h. Intra-rater reliability
i. Predictive validity
j. Test/re-test reliability

Lead in

Select one property each that the following imaginary rating scales have:

Scales

1. Subjects with an DSM-IV diagnosis of a major depressive disorder have much higher scores on the YDR than subjects without a major depressive disorder.
2. Subjects with OCD are rated using a new scale, the COCDS, together with an older, well-validated scale. Scores on the two scales are strongly correlated.
3. In a multi-centre treatment study, research assessors from the different sites listen to a random sample of tape-recorded assessments carried out by their colleagues. They score the subjects' anxiety symptomatology using the AAA based on their colleagues' assessments, blinded to their colleagues' scores. All research assessors give very similar AAA scores for each interview.
4. After suicide attempts, assessing psychiatrists rated each patient using the REPEAT. All patients were followed up over 6 months. Subjects with high scores on the REPEAT were much more likely to make a further suicide attempt than those with low scores.
5. A new self-report questionnaire for adolescent depression, the ADQ, has questions covering in detail emotional symptoms, cognitive symptoms, biological symptoms (including headaches and stomach aches) and behavioural symptoms.

Answers

15.1 Alternatives to standard statistical procedures

1-e. Mann–Whitney test.
2-j. Wilcoxon signed-rank test.
3-d. Kruskall–Wallis test.
4-f. Spearman's test.
5-a. Fisher's exact test.

15.2 Biases

1-h. Recall bias. In case–control studies, cases may be more likely to be aware of the possible risk factors they have been exposed to in the past.
2-a. Attrition bias.
3-b. Berkson's bias – or admission rate bias/paradox – refers to when the exposure of interest increases admission rates, and can cause problems when recruiting in-patients in case–control studies.
4-d. Information bias. Knowledge of the results of the screen may affect the diagnostic assessment (or vice-versa).
5-i. Selection bias. Knowing which treatment group patients will go into (even if allocation is truly random) may affect how the recruiter discusses the trial with potential subjects, and therefore whether they go into the study. The treatment groups may then be unbalanced.

15.3 Characteristics of a good test

1-h. Standardisation.
2-f. Sensitivity.
3-e. Reliability.
4-g. Specificity.
5-j. Validity.

15.4 Multivariate statistical procedures

1-g. MANOVA.
2-j. RMANOVA.
3-f. Multiple regression analysis.
4-e. Logistic regression analysis.
5-c. Factor analysis.

15.5 Statistical concepts

1-i. Predictive validity (Jacoby & Oppenheimer-85).

2-h. Known group validity.

3-d. Criterion validity.

4-a. Concurrent validity.

5-c. Convergent and divergent validity.

15.6 Statistical tests

1-h. Multiple logistic regression. Multiple regression allows investigating the associations between several putative risk factors and an outcome of interest. When investigating the possible effects of each risk factor, all other risk factors are controlled for. If the outcome of interest is binary, i.e. yes/no, diagnosis present/absent, multiple logistic regression is used.

2-c. Chi-squared – used for comparing counts, e.g. number of cases, number of patients recovered between two or more groups. If values are very small in one sub-group, Fisher's exact test may have to be used.

3-b. ANOVA. When comparing more than two groups, the first analysis must be to find out if there is any difference across the groups. This is ANOVA (analysis of variance) if data are normally distributed, Kruskal–Wallis if non-normal.

4-f. Mann-Whitney test. In comparing a continuous outcome measure between two groups, the Mann–Whitney test must be used if data is not normally distributed. If transforming the data, e.g. by log or square root, gives normally-distributed data, then parametric statistical methods, e.g. Student's t-test, can be used.

5-a. ANCOVA – used to compare outcomes if two groups differ at baseline. It is valid only if data is normally distributed and if baseline and final measures correlate. It is a type of multiple regression, and not a type of ANOVA.

15.7 Study designs

1-d. Cost utility study. They take into account differences in the quality and quantity of life. This is often measured as Quality Adjusted Life Years (QALYs) as well as in costs between different treatments.

2-f. Ecological study. The group rather than the individual is the unit of measurement.

3-j. Retrospective cohort study. Cohort studies start with cohorts exposed or not to a factor of interest, and are followed up to see the difference in outcomes of interest between these groups. They can be prospective, i.e. cohorts found and investigated at the start of the study, or retrospective, i.e. historical cohorts found and exposure status at start investigated.

4-g. Open-label RCT. All parties know the treatment the subjects are receiving.

5-c. Cost-effectiveness study.

15.8 Treatment effects

1-a. Absolute benefit increase. The absolute numerical difference between the rates of good outcome between experimental and control participants in a trial (Lawrie-111).

2-i. Relative risk. The risk of the event in question in the experimental group divided by the risk of the same event in controls.

3-b. Absolute risk reduction. The absolute numerical difference between the rates of adverse outcomes in the control and experimental groups.

4-j. Relative risk reduction. The percent reduction in events in an experimental group compared with controls.

5-e. Number needed to treat. The inverse of absolute benefit increase. The number of people who need to be given the active treatment to prevent one event that would have occurred had they been in the control group.

15.9 Univariate statistics

1-j. Student's *t*-test.

2-a. ANOVA.

3-i. Pearson's product-moment correlation coefficient.

4-b. Chi-square test.

5-d. Kappa coefficient.

15.10 Validity

1-a. Criterion validity. Strictly speaking, criterion validity refers to the comparison with a known quantity, such as height. In practice, the term is often used to refer to the comparison between an outcome scale and an absolute diagnosis.

2-b. Concurrent validity – the agreement with another scale, which has itself been shown to be valid.

3-g. Inter-rater reliability – the degree of concordance between the scores given by different raters.

4-i. Predictive validity – the agreement between a present measurement and one in the future.

5-c. Content validity – refers to when a scale covers all of the important subject matter.

References

In the answers, the numbers that follow the abbreviations of the references indicate the page numbers.

1. Anderson I, Reid I. (2002) *Fundamentals of Clinical Psychopharmacology.* London: Taylor & Francis (**Anderson & Reid**)

2. Arseneault L. *et al* (2004) Causal association between cannabis and psychosis: examination of the evidence. Br J Psychiatry 184: 110–117 (Arseneault *et al* 2004)

3. Barrett P. *et al* (2004) Cognitive-behavioural family treatment of childhood obsessive-compulsive disorder: a controlled trial. JAACAP 43: 46–62 (Barrett *et al* 2004)

4. Goodwin GM. (2003) Evidence Based Guidelines for Treating Bipolar Disorder: Recommendations from the British Association for Psychopharmacology. http://www.bap.org.uk (**BAP-B**)

5. Anderson IM, Nutt DJ, Deakin JFW. (2000). Evidence based Guidelines for treating depressive disorders with antidepressants: A Revision of the 1993 BAP Guidelines. http://www.bap.org.uk (**BAP-D**)

6. Bazire S. (2003) *Psychotropic Drug Directory (2003–4)* Salisbury: Fivepin (**Bazire**)

7. Bion, WR (1959) *Experiences in Group and Other Papers.* New York: Basic Books (**Bion**)

8. Bleuler E. (1912) (English edn. 1950). *Dementia praecox or the group of schizophrenias.* New York: International University Press (**Bleuler**)

9. Bloch S. (1998) *Introduction to the Psychotherapies.* 3rd edn. Oxford: Oxford University Press (**Bloch**)

10. *British National Formulary, 47.* London: BMA and RPSGB, March 2004 (**BNF47**)

11. Brown GW, Harris TO. (1978) *Social Origins of Depression.* London: Tavistock (**Brown & Harris**)

12. Callicott JH. *et al* (2000) Physiological dysfunction of the dorsolateral prefrontal cortex in schizophrenia revisited. Cereb Cortex, 10: 1078–92 (Callicott *et al* 2000)

13. Chick J, Cantweel R. (1994) *Seminars in Alcohol and Drug Misuse.* London: Gaskell (**Chick & Cantweel**)

14. The UK Creutzfeldt–Jakob Disease Surveillance Unit. http://www.cjd.ed.ac.uk (**CJD**)

15. Edwards G, Marshall JE, Cook C. (2003) *The Treatment of Drinking Problems.* 4th edn., Cambridge: Cambridge University Press (**Edwards**)

16. Wright P, Stern J, Phelan M. (2000) *Core Psychiatry.* London: Saunders (**Core**)

17. Johnstone EC *et al* (2004) *Companion to Psychiatric Studies.* 7th edn., Edinburgh: Churchill Livingstone (**CPS7**)

18. Sadock, BJ, Sadock VA. (2000) *Kaplan & Sadock's Comprehensive Textbook of Psychiatry.* 7th edn., Philadelphia: Williams & Wilkins (**CTP7**)

19. Davies JM. *et al* (2003) A meta-analysis of the efficacy of second-generation antipsychotics. Arch Gen Psychiatry, 60 :553–64 (Davies *et al* 2003)

20. Department of Health. http://www.dh.gov.uk (**DH**)

21. Di Rocco A, Werner P. (1999) Hypothesis on the pathogenesis of vacuolar myelopathy, dementia, and peripheral neuropathy in AIDS. J Neurol Neurosurg Psychiatry, 66:554 (Di Ricco & Werner, 1999)

22. Dierks T. *et al* (1999) Activation of Heschl's gyrus during auditory hallucinations. Neuron, 22: 615–621 (Dierks *et al* 1999)

23. American Psychiatric Association. (1994) *Diagnostic and Statistical Manual of Mental Disorders*. 4th edn., Washington, DC: APA (**DSM-IV**)

24. Freeman CP. (1995). ECT Handbook: The 2nd report of the Royal College of Psychiatrists Special Committee on ECT. Council Report CR39 (**ECT**)

25. Enoch D, Ball H. (2001) *Uncommon Psychiatric Syndromes*. 4th edn., London: Arnold (**Enoch & Ball**)

26. Murray R, Hill P, McGuffin P. (1997) *Essentials of Postgraduate Psychiatry*. 3rd edn., Cambridge: Cambridge University Press (**EPP3**)

27. Stein S, Haigh R, Stein J. (1999) *Essentials of Psychotherapy*. Oxford: Butterworth-Heinemann (**EPS**)

28. Hamilton M. (1974) *Fish's Clinical Psychopathology*. Bristol: Wright (**Fish**)

29. Fitzgerald M, Folan-Curran J. (2002) *Clinical Anatomy and Related Neuroscience*. Philadelphia: Saunders (**Fitzgerald & Folan-Curran**)

30. Fraser W, Kerr M. (2003) *Seminars in the Psychiatry of Learning Disabilities*. 2nd edn., London: Gaskell (**Fraser & Kerr**)

31. Goodman R, Scott S. (1997) *Child Psychiatry*. Oxford: Blackwell Science (**Goodman & Scott**)

32. Goodyer, IM. *et al* (1996) Adrenal secretion during major depression in 8- to 16-year-olds, I. Altered diurnal rhythms in salivary cortisol and dehydroepiandrosterone (DHEA) at presentation. Psychol Med, 26: 245–56 (Goodyer *et al* 1996)

33. Green MF. (2001) *Schizophrenia Revealed*. New York: Norton (**Green**)

34. Gross R. (2001) *Psychology. The Science of Mind and Behaviour*. 4th edn., London: Hodder & Stoughton (**Gross**)

35. Hafner H. *et al* (1999) Depression, negative symptoms, social stagnation and social decline in the early course of schizophrenia. Acta Psychiatr Scand, 100: 105–18 (Hafner *et al* 1999)

36. Hay PJ, Bacaltchuk J. (2004) Psychotherapy for bulimia nervosa and binging. Cochrane Library 2004; 1 (Hay & Bacaltchuk 2004)

37. Atkinson RL. *et al*. (2000) *Hilgard's Introduction to Psychology*. 13th edn., Fort Worth: Harcourt College Publishers (**Hilgard**)

38. Hoch P, Polatin P. (1949) Pseudoneurotic forms of schizophrenia. Psychiatry Quarterly, 23: 248–256 (Hoch & Polatin 1949)

39. Hodges JR. (1994) *Cognitive Assessment for Clinicians*. Oxford: Oxford University Press (**Hodges**)

40. World Health Organisation (1992). *The ICD-10 Classification of Mental and Behavioural Disorders*. Geneva: WHO (**ICD-10**)

41. Jacoby R, Oppenheimer C. (2002) *Psychiatry in the Elderly*. 3rd edn., Oxford: Oxford University Press (**Jacoby & Oppenheimer**)

42. Kapur S. *et al* (2000) Relationship between dopamine (D(2) occupancy, clinical response, and side effects: a double-blind PET study of first-episode schizophrenia. Am J Psychiatry, 157: 514–20 (Kapur *et al* 2000)

43. Kasanin J. (1933). The acute schizoaffective psychoses. Am J Psychiatry, 13: 97–126 (Kasanin 1933)

44. Katona CLE, Livingston G. (2002) *Drug Treatment in Old Age Psychiatry*. London: Martin Dunitz (**Katona & Livingston**)

45. Kemp R. *et al* (1998) Randomised controlled trial of compliance therapy. 18-month follow-up. Br J Psychiatry, 172: 413–19 (Kemp *et al* 1998)

46. King DJ. (1995) *Seminars in Clinical Psychopharmacology.* London: Gaskell (**King**)

47. Kaplan HI, Sadock BJ, Sadock VA. (2000) *Pocket Handbook of Psychiatric Drug Treatment.* 3rd edn., Philadelphia: Lippincott Williams and Wilkins (**KSDT**)

48. Sadock BJ, Sadock VA. (2002) *Kaplan & Sadock's Synopsis of Psychiatry.* 9th edn., Philadelphia: Lippincott Williams & Wilkins (**KSP9**)

49. Kuipers E. *et al* (1997) London-East Anglia randomised controlled trial of cognitive-behavioural therapy for psychosis. I: effects of the treatment phase. Br J Psychiatry, 171: 319–27 (Kuipers *et al* 1997)

50. Langfeldt G. (1960) Diagnosis and prognosis of schizophrenia. Proceedings of the Royal Society of Medicine, 53: 1047–1052 (Langfeldt 1960)

51. Lawlor B. (2001) *Revision Psychiatry.* Dublin: MedMedia (**Lawlor**)

52. Lawrie SM, McIntosh A, Rao S. (2000) *Critical Appraisal for Psychiatry.* Edinburgh: Churchill Livingstone (**Lawrie**)

53. Lishman WA. (1997) *Organic Psychiatry.* 3rd edn., Oxford: Blackwell Science (**Lishman**)

54. McClellan JM, Werry JS. (2003) Evidence-based treatments in child and adolescent psychiatry: an inventory. J Am Acad Child Adolesc Psychiatry, 42: 1388–400 (McClellan & Werry 2003)

55. McKenna PJ. (1997) *Schizophrenia and Related Syndromes.* Hove: Psychology Press (**McKenna**)

56. Medicines and Healthcare products Regulatory Agency. http://www.mhra.gov.uk (**MHRA**)

57. Mayer-Gross W. (1924) *Selbstschilderungen der Verwirrtheit; die oneirode Erlebnisform.* Monographien aus dem Gesamtgebiete der Neurologie und Psychiatrie, Berlin, H. 42 (Mayer-Gross 1924)

58. Moreno ZT. (1975) A survey of psychodramatic techniques. Group Psychotherapy, 12: 5–14 (Moreno, 1975)

59. Mortensen PB. *et al* (1999) Effects of family history and place and season of birth on the risk of schizophrenia. N Engl J Med, 340: 603–8 (Mortensen *et al* 1999)

60. Taylor D, Paton C, Kerwin R. (2003) *Maudsley Prescribing Guidelines.* 7th edn., London: Martin Dunitz (**MPG7**)

61. Mufson L. *et al* (1999) Efficacy of interpersonal psychotherapy for depressed adolescents. Arch Gen Psychiatry, 56: 573–9 (Mufson *et al* 1999)

62. Niemi LT. *et al* (2003) Childhood developmental abnormalities in schizophrenia: evidence from high-risk studies. Schizophrenia Res, 60: 239–258 (Niemi *et al* 2003)

63. Hale AS, Malhi G, Matharoo MS. (2000) *Neurology for Psychiatrists.* London: Taylor & Francis (**NFP**)

64. National Institute for Clinical Excellence. NICE guidelines. http://www.nice.org.uk (**NICE**)

65. Gelder MG, Andreasen NC, Lopez-Ibor JJ. (2000) *New Oxford Textbook of Psychiatry.* Oxford: Oxford University Press (**NOTP**)

66. O'Brien, J, Barber B. (2000) Neuroimaging in dementia and depression. Advan Psychiatr Treat, 6: 109–19 (O'Brien & Barber, 2000)

67. Ødegärd Ø. (1932) Emigration and insanity. Acta Psych Scand, Suppl 4 (Ødegärd 1932)

68. Hope RA. *et al.* (1998) *Oxford Handbook of Clinical Medicine,* 4th edn., Oxford: Oxford University Press (**OM4**)

69. Cowen P, Gelder M, Mayou R. (2001) *Shorter Oxford Textbook of Psychiatry.* 4th edn., Oxford: Oxford University Press (**OTP4**)

70. Parsey RV, Mann JJ. (2003) Applications of positron emission tomography in psychiatry. Semin Nucl Med, 33: 129–35 (Parsey & Mann 2003)

71. Kandel E, Schwartz J, Jessel T. (2000) *Principles of Neural Science.* New York: McGraw-Hill (**PNS**)

72. Prochaska JO, DiClemente CC (1986) Towards a comprehensive model of change. In *Treating addictive behaviours: Process of change.* (eds WR Miller, and N Heather) pp3–27. New York: Plenum Press (**Prochaska & DiClemente**)

73. Rabins PV. *et al* (1991) Cortical magnetic resonance imaging changes in elderly inpatients with major depression. Am J Psychiatry, 148: 617–20 (Rabins *et al* 1991)

74. Rutter M, Taylor E. (2002) *Child and Adolescent Psychiatry.* 4th edn., Oxford: Blackwell Science (**Rutter & Taylor**)

75. Jacobson JL, Jacobson AM. (2001) *Psychiatric Secrets.* 2nd edn., Philadelphia: Hanley & Belfus 2001 (**Secrets**)

76. Sims A. (2000) *Symptoms in the Mind.* 2nd edn., London: Saunders (**Sims**)

77. Smith RL. *et al* (1999) Mechanism of tolerance development to 2,5-dimethoxy-4-iodoamphetamine in rats: down-regulation of the 5-HT2A, but not 5-HT2C, receptor. Psychopharmacology (Berl). 144: 248–54 (Smith *et al* 1999)

78. Spencer MD. *et al,* (2002) First hundred cases of variant Creutzfeldt–Jakob disease: retrospective case note review of early psychiatric and neurological features. BMJ, 324 (7352): 479–82 (Spencer *et al* 2002)

79. Stein G, Wilkinson G. (1998) *Seminars in General Adult Psychiatry.* London: Gaskell (**Stein & Wilkinson**)

80. Travis MJ. *et al* (1998) 5-HT2A receptor blockade in patients with schizophrenia treated with risperidone or clozapine. A SPET study using the novel 5-HT2A ligand 123I-5-I-R-91150. Br J Psychiatry, 173: 236–41 (Travis *et al* 1998)

81. Ucok A. *et al* (2004) Duration of untreated psychosis may predict acute treatment response in first-episode schizophrenia. J Psychiatr Res, 38: 163–8 (Ucok *et al* 2004)

82. Yalom ID. (1994) *The Theory & Practice of Group Psychotherapy.* 4th edn., New York: Basic Books (**Yalom**)

83. Yudofsky SC, Hales RE. (2002) *Textbook of Neuropsychiatry and Clinical Neurosciences.* Arlington, VA: American Psychiatric Publishing (**Yudofsky & Hales**)

84. Wykes T. *et al* (2003) Are the effects of cognitive remediation therapy (CRT) durable? Results from an exploratory trial in schizophrenia. Schizophr Res. 61: 163–74 (Wykes *et al* 2003)